descriptive medical electronics & instrumentation

Terence Karselis, M.T. (ASCP)
Assistant Professor,
Department of Medical Technology,
State University of New York at Buffalo

Charles B. Slack, Inc.　·　New Jersey

Library of Congress Catalog Number: 73-77964
ISBN: 0-913590-05-3

FIRST PRINTING, MARCH 1973

To Lil and Ed,
who made it possible,
and to Judy,
who made it worthwhile

foreword

Medical electronics and instrumentation can no longer be called a new part of today's medicine. Over the past fifteen years the dramatic accomplishments in this field have revolutionized not only hospital laboratories, but also intensive care and coronary care units to the point that in almost every corner of today's rapidly expanding health care centers, some form of electronic instrumentation can be found. For those individuals required to work with the sophisticated equipment in this rapidly growing technology, a knowledge of basic electronics and instrumentation is invaluable. To utilize a medical electronic device to its full capability, its operator must not only know *How?* the device works, but he must also have some idea of *Why?*

This volume is intended to help a broad spectrum of allied health students, including medical technologists, physical therapists, and bioengineering technologists, etc., as well as nurses and medical students to achieve an introduction to the *Why?* of basic electronics and medical instrumentation. In addition, it will provide them with a cross-sectional view of the electronic "tools" used by their various colleagues on the health care team.

The material presented in this book is an outgrowth of lectures which I prepared for a one semester course in *Basic Electronics for Medical Technologists* at the State University of New York at Buffalo. The need for such a broad-based descriptive introductory text became obvious when an increasing number of chemistry, biology and physical therapy students were attracted to the course.

To appeal to a wide spectrum of allied health workers, with their varied backgrounds and interests, a descriptive or "understanding" approach has been used to present the material. To find the information useful a potential reader need be familiar with only a few basic principles of algebra, chemistry, and physics.

As one consequence of using a descriptive approach, it has been necessary to omit or simplify some of the facts, concepts, and theory that others may deem important. I take complete and full responsibility for such liberties and apologize to my more informed readers.

The material is divided into four parts. *Part One* covers basic electronics up to and including integrated circuits; *Part Two* is a survey of the electronics involved in analytical instrumentation; *Part Three* deals with diagnostic instrumentation and therapeutic devices; and *Part Four* is concerned with safety.

The many circuit and block diagrams presented in the text are intended to be illustrative examples and not constructional information; consequently component values, etc., are not indicated.

I gratefully acknowledge the outstanding aid and support of many individuals in the preparation of this work: Sylvia Kurland, Agnes Loesch, Bertha Glaberman, and Pat O'Connor for preparing the manuscript; Dr. John V. Fopeano and Sara Marie Cicarelli for planting the seed; and my students who by their enthusiasm kept the idea growing. I am also grateful to the manufacturers and armed services who supplied illustrative material.

Special thanks are due to my wife and family for their enthusiastic support, prompting, and understanding.

Terence C. Karselis

contents

thyratrons; cathode ray tubes (CRT); photo-tubes; storage cathode ray tubes

SECTION II
CLINICAL ANALYTICAL INSTRUMENTATION
(Chapters 17-20)

transducers, photo-transistors); nuclear transducers—radioactive energy transducers; flow rate transducers (electromagnetic detectors, thermal detectors, sonic detectors, ionization detectors)

SECTION III
MEDICAL ELECTRONICS AND BIOENGINEERING
(Chapters 21-28)

preface

During the past few years, curricula revision has been one of the hallmarks of the educational programs at all levels for the allied health professions and occupations. These changes have been essential to respond to the expanding professional role in these fields, to the development of more sophisticated techniques, and to evolving technological advancements. Research in bioelectronics, instrumentation, and automation has already exerted a profound influence on the ways in which diagnosis, analysis, and health care services are to be delivered by allied health personnel.

It was propitious for this school that a member of its faculty in the Department of Medical Technology was keenly interested in the expanding relationship between electronics and allied health. This text is an outgrowth of an electronics course that was developed several years ago, and its presentation has been received with enthusiasm by medical technology students. With imagination and dedication, the author has nurtured his original concepts into a manuscript and core course that now appeals to the needs of both health and basic science students from many disciplines.

The patients we serve will be the ultimate benefactors of the insight and wisdom which developed this book so that allied health students might be in a position to deliver more effective health care because of a clearer understanding of the changing instrumentation and automation in these specialized fields of service.

J. Warren Perry, Ph.D.
Dean, School of Health Related Professions
Professor, Health Sciences Administration
State University of New York at Buffalo
17 Diefendorf Annex
Buffalo, New York, 1970

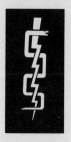

SECTION 1

basic electricity
and electronics

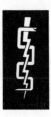 basic theory and definitions

CHAPTER 1

This book is by no means meant to prepare anyone to be a qualified electronics technician. It is designed, however, to build a background in those areas of electronics which are commonly found in clinical instruments and associated devices, albeit at the expense of other information usually found in more conventional texts.

The material is organized on a practical or descriptive rather than an analytical level. This arrangement was chosen for two reasons: (1) the time available for students or workers in the health professions to familiarize themselves with this subject is too short to cover the required subject matter in analytical depth; and (2) the author's goal is to assist the worker to understand the operating principles of any instrument he may use in the future, *not* to teach him to design or repair them extensively. Simple trouble-shooting, although discussed, is not a primary objective. To reach this "understanding" level, it is not necessary to analyze circuit problems such as phase relationships, or to calculate values of mutual inductance. It will suffice to know *how* phase differences are produced, *what* mutual inductance is, and *how* it is used.

After reading this volume, it is hoped that the worker will be able to approach an unfamiliar instrument with confidence and, by use of operational handbooks and circuit diagrams, gain a firm understanding of its operating principles.

Simple trouble-shooting (finding defective components in an instrument by logical step-by-step methods) is an art. It requires three things: (1) that the worker clearly understand the functional subunits or areas of the instrument; (2) that he know or can find out, by reference to the manufacturer's manual, the inputs and outputs of each subunit; and (3) most important of all, that he be capable of using test equipment to detect these inputs and outputs. The most common piece of test equipment is the **VOM** (*V*olt-*O*hm-*M*illiammeter) sometimes called a **multimeter**. This is an instrument capable of measuring **voltage, current,** and **resistance** (the three basic units of electrical activity). To use this device effectively requires some analytical knowledge. Simple calculations involving Ohm's law will therefore be included in a later chapter which will enable the worker to perform such analysis.

SAFETY

The most overworked and yet the most ignored word in use today is *safety*. Wherever we go we are given precautions and told what "not to do," etc.—and yet these instructions are usually ignored. To be different, let us use another term: *respect*. This is the term with which all prospective workers with electronics should identify. Electricity can harm us or work for us; it should therefore be respected. In so doing the worker will find himself naturally following precautions and consequently working more safely.

Electronic Safety Rules

By combining respect for electricity with a few fundamental rules good work habits can be developed and the possibility of a serious accident decreased. The following rules should be well studied and obeyed.

1. Keep one hand clear when handling energized parts or wiring.
2. Make visual checks of wiring for short circuits, before applying power.
3. Never handle energized electronic equipment while in contact with a damp surface.
4. Energized electrical parts are potentially dangerous. Make sure surfaces are insulated if they must be handled.
5. Do not wear loose jewelry around electronic equipment in operation.
6. When making measurements with power on, keep one hand clear.
7. Do not probe hot circuits indiscriminately. Use only

approved test equipment. All equipment should be properly grounded.

8. Never work alone on high voltage electronic equipment.
9. Use only insulated tools.
10. Use large amounts of common sense.

By following these simple rules and respecting (but not fearing) electricity the worker will find himself using and handling instruments with more confidence than he had previously thought possible.

BASIC TERMS AND DEFINITIONS

The three fundamental entities upon which the theories of electricity and electronics rest are **voltage, current,** and **resistance.** We will define and briefly discuss each in turn; however, it will simplify matters if we first consider a few other definitions which relate to these fundamentals.

Free electrons are those electrons, loosely bound to an atom, which require only small amounts of additional energy to enable them to "break free" from their orbits and pass to another atom. Within many materials a few of these electrons are at all times "drifting" through its molecular structure in random fashion.

Conductors are those materials that have a relatively large number of free electrons, thereby making them a good substance through which to pass an electric current.

Insulators (or nonconductors) are those materials that have relatively few free electrons and consequently poor conductors of electric current.

With these three definitions clearly in mind, we can now progress on to *voltage, current,* and *resistance.*

Voltage/EMF/Difference of Potential: Voltage is defined as *the difference in charge or potential energy existing between two points due to an unbalanced electron population at those two points.* For example, imagine we could hold ten atoms of some material in each hand, and that in the right hand we have five *extra* electrons while in the left hand we are five electrons *short.* The atoms in both hands will be charged. The right hand has a *negative* charge (-) due to its excess electrons, while the left hand has a *positive* charge (+) due to its deficiency of electrons. This *difference in potential energy* can be used to produce a current flow; hence it is also termed **electromotive force (EMF)**. We will examine this action in the definition of electrical current.

Current flow is defined as *the movement or migration of free electrons through a conductor due to the influence of a difference of potential existing across the conductor*. Once more, remembering the analogy of holding atoms in our hands, we will assume the same situation of a negatively charged right hand and a positively charged left hand. This time, however, we will connect a material which contains many free electrons (a conductor) between the right and left hands. The moment such a connection is made, the following reaction takes place:

1. An electron passes from the conductor into the left hand, which is deficient in electrons.
2. This creates a deficiency at the left end of the conductor. This deficiency is filled by a chain reaction of electrons moving (in a "musical chairs" fashion) all the way through the material until the deficiency has been reflected to the other (or right) end of the material.
3. One of the extra electrons from the right hand is then injected into this deficiency. (Figure 1-1 illustrates this

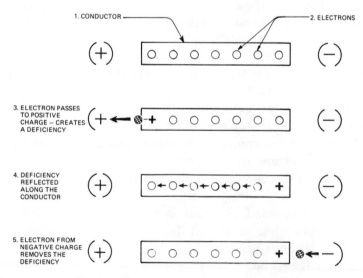

Fig. 1-1: Electron movement in a conductor

sequence of events.) This directed movement of free electrons constitutes *current flow*.

Resistance refers to the opposition, inherent in any material, to electric current. The amount of current that flows through a conductor is directly proportional to the number of free electrons available in the conductor; therefore, the amount of resistance shown by the material is *inversely* proportional to the number of free electrons available. The *more* free electrons there are to carry current, the *lower* the resistance; the *less* electrons, the *higher* the resistance.

There are no perfect conductors or nonconductors; consequently, there is no such thing as absolute zero resistance—there exists some opposition to current flow in all materials. The relationship between conductor and insulator or nonconductor is a relative one, determined by the molecular structure of the substance in question. This gives rise to the term **resistivity**.

Silver is arbitrarily given the value of 1.00. The actual resistance of a piece of any material depends on its shape and size; the length and cross-sectional area of any piece of material must be taken into account when evaluating its resistance. The following are the relative resistivities of some common metals.

Silver	(Ag)	= 1.00	Aluminum	(Al)	= 1.8
Copper	(Cu)	= 1.08	Lead	(Pb)	= 13.5
Gold	(Au)	= 1.4	Platinum	(Pt)	= 7.0

The resistance of any substance is sensitive to temperature change; each material has its own **temperature coefficient.** In general, resistance *increases* with an *increase* in temperature. A material that acts in this way is said to have a *positive* temperature coefficient. Carbon is unique in that it has a *negative* temperature coefficient; with an *increase* in temperature, its resistance *decreases*.

Gases are usually considered to have high resistances; they can, however, conduct current when ionized. Ionization releases electrons for current flow and it may be brought about in two ways:

1. Bombarding the gas with energy (light or x-rays);
2. Placing the gas in a high energy electrostatic field.

The ionization of gases is employed in the design of many instruments, from power supplies to scintillation counter detectors.

TYPES OF CURRENT FLOW

The three basic types of current flow can be defined by referring to **polarity**, or direction of flow, and **magnitude**.

1. A **direct current** (DC) is one in which *magnitude and polarity remain fixed with relation to time.*
2. An **alternating current** (AC) *reverses polarity* periodically and is constantly *changing in magnitude.*
3. A **pulsating direct current** has *fixed polarity* but its *magnitude varies.*

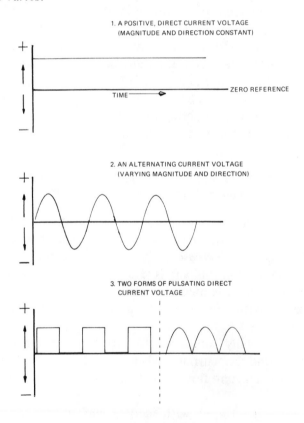

Fig. 1-2: *Current waveforms*

MEASURING DEVICES

The following paragraphs are meant to serve as an introduction to the most common electrical measuring devices. These will be studied in more detail in a later chapter.

Before progressing further, the term *polarity* should be defined. **Polarity** refers to the negative or positive *direction* of a current or voltage. It can also, in many instances, be used to refer to points in a circuit as being relatively positive or negative with respect to each other. For instance, **to observe polarity** means that when a test instrument is connected to a circuit, the negative or common lead (usually black) is connected to a negative point, while the positive lead (usually red) is connected to a positive point. This allows current to flow in the proper direction through the test instrument. Figure 1-2 demonstrates types of current flow and the concept of polarity.

Voltmeter
(An Electrical Pressure Sampler)

A **voltmeter** can be imagined as a pressure sampler since it measures the electrical pressure between two points in a circuit. A voltmeter then performs the function its name implies: it measures voltage.

NOTE: A voltmeter is connected to the circuit **in parallel, never in series** *(Figure 1-3). The concepts of series and*

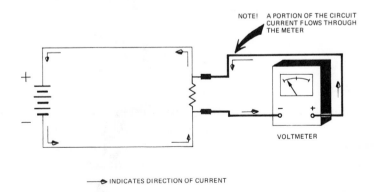

Fig. 1-3: Method of connecting a voltmeter to a circuit

parallel will be covered in the next chapter. When measuring a DC voltage, be sure to observe polarity (black lead to negative—red lead to positive). When measuring an AC voltage, polarity need not be observed (it is compensated for within the meter).

Ammeter
(An Electrical Flow Meter)

An **ammeter** can be envisioned as a flow meter since it samples the current flowing through the circuit. An ammeter (or milli-ammeter) must be connected to the circuit in series and, before any attachments are made, power must first be turned off. Power is reapplied after the meter is connected into the circuit. When direct current flow is measured, *polarity must be observed.* Figure 1-4 shows the correct way to hook up an ammeter.

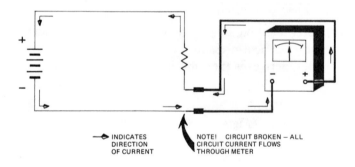

INDICATES DIRECTION OF CURRENT

NOTE! CIRCUIT BROKEN – ALL CIRCUIT CURRENT FLOWS THROUGH METER

Fig. 1-4: Method of connecting an ammeter to a circuit

Ohmmeter

An **ohmmeter** is used to measure resistance and to check for "shorted" or "open" circuits. *It is used only when power to the circuit under test has been removed.* When resistance is to be measured, one end of the component under test must be disconnected from the circuit. Figure 1-5 shows the correct method for measuring resistance. The ohmmeter supplies its own power from an internal battery.

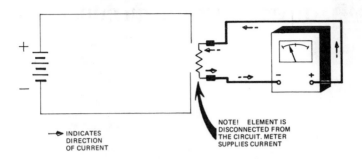

NOTE! ELEMENT IS DISCONNECTED FROM THE CIRCUIT. METER SUPPLIES CURRENT

INDICATES DIRECTION OF CURRENT

Fig 1-5: Method of connecting an ohmmeter

NOTE: When measuring voltage or current, be sure to start with the highest range of the meter and work down until you reach the setting that gives the most sensitive reading.

Example: To measure an unknown voltage with a voltmeter that has three ranges of 0-10 volts, 0-100 volts, and 0-1000 volts, we start by using the 0-1000 volt range. Why? Suppose the unknown value is 9 volts. On the 1000 volts range, this will not cause much of a deflection (about to the 10 volt mark). We then switch volts range. Once again, we will see only a small deflection (about to the 10 volts mark). We then switch to the 10 volts range. On this range we will see almost a full scale deflection, giving the most accurate reading.

There are two reasons for this precaution. If we need to measure an unknown voltage (it is 300 volts but we have no way of knowing this until it is measured), and we start on the 0-10 volt range, the moment the meter is connected, the indicator needle will jump off scale and the instrument may possibly be ruined since it only requires 10 volts to give a full scale deflection at that range. This first reason is obviously based on *Safety First* rules.

The second reason is based on common sense. A 9 volt value causes more deflection and consequently may be read with more sensitivity on the 0-10 volt range than on the 0-100 volt range.

direct current circuit laws

CHAPTER 2

OHM'S LAW

Between voltage, current, and resistance there exists an interesting relationship first discovered by George Simon Ohm, a German physicist (1787-1854). He published his findings in 1827 and we now know them as **Ohm's Law**. This fundamental law of electricity states:

> **THE CURRENT IN AN ELECTRICAL CONDUCTOR IS DIRECTLY PROPORTIONAL TO THE VOLTAGE BETWEEN THE ENDS OF THE CONDUCTOR AND INVERSELY PROPORTIONAL TO THE RESISTANCE.**

The relationship between the three values can be easily seen, since an increase in pressure will obviously give an increased flow (opposition remaining constant) while an increase in opposition will result in a decreased flow (pressure remaining constant).

Before discussing the equations derived from Ohm's law, we should first define the **unit values** of current, voltage, and resistance.

1. **Current** is defined as *the rate of movement of free electrons through a conductor.* Since electrons are minute particles and we must have some convenient term by which to express units of current flow, we designate the charge of a mass of 6.28×10^{18} electrons as a **coulomb.** We further state that *a charge of one coulomb passing a given point per second is one ampere of current flow.* In short, current is measured by the rate at which electrons flow.

2. **The unit of voltage** (or electromotive force—EMF) is the **volt**, defined as *the difference of potential required to maintain a current flow of one ampere through a resistance of one ohm.*
3. **The unit of resistance** is the **ohm**. A conductor has a resistance of one ohm if a voltage across it of one volt results in a current through it of one ampere. Resistance can also be calculated on the basis of resistivity, length, and cross-sectional area as follows:

$$R = \frac{\rho L}{A}$$

where ρ = resistivity (resistance between opposite faces of a 1 cm cube of the specific material
L = length in centimeters
A = cross-section area (cm^2)
R = resistance in ohms

Symbols

The symbol for voltage is E; for current, I; and for resistance, R.

Units

The units of voltage, current flow, and resistance may be given in many varied forms, a number of which follow:

Unit	Symbol	Abbreviations	Multiple Units			
			x 10^{+3}	x 10^{+6}	x 10^{-3}	10^{-6}
Volt	E	V	KV (kilovolt)	MV (megavolt)	mv (millivolt)	μv (microvolt)
Ampere	I	amps	—	—	ma (milliamps)	μa (microamps)
Ohm	R	Ω (omega)	KΩ (kilohm)	MΩ (megohm)	—	—

Ohm's Law may be given as an equation in any of these three forms:

$$I = E \div R$$
$$R = E \div I$$
$$E = I \times R$$

The following memory aid will help us remember Ohm's Law. To obtain the formula for an unknown, place your finger over the symbol for the required quantity; the formula is then revealed.

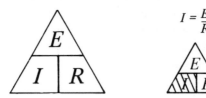

$$I = \frac{E}{R}$$

POWER

When current flows through a conductor, a certain amount of energy is dissipated as heat (and sometimes light) into the environment around the conductor. We use resistances in circuits to develop required values of voltage and current flow; these values determine the rate of energy dissipation. The rate at which energy is dissipated is called **power** and is measured in **watts**. It is given the symbol P, and can be calculated by the formula:

$$P = I^2 R$$

The power dissipated by resistances is detrimental for two reasons: (1) it represents lost energy, and (2) it increases the temperature of the equipment.

Two other formulas are available for calculating power:

$$P = EI \quad \text{and} \quad P = E^2 \div R$$

HOLES AND ELECTRONS

It is likely that at some time in the future you will be faced with a puzzling situation: one worker may state that current flows from negative to positive poles, and another worker states that current flows from positive to negative poles. In which direction *does* current flow? To solve this enigma we must look at what happens in a conductor when a voltage is impressed across it. If we look at a single atom at the first instant the difference in potential is applied, we will see an electron pulled free in the direction of the positive voltage. As soon as this occurs, we have, for an instant in time, a **positive-negative charge pair** in existence—the electron representing the negative charge; the "hole" (or absence of an electron) in the atom representing the positive charge. (This generation of a positive-negative charge pair—or "hole" electron pair—is important in the theory of semiconductors.)

Referring to Figure 2-1, we can see that, as electrons move through a conductor in one direction, there are apparent migration of "holes" or *positive charges* in the opposite direction. (It is this positive charge movement that is sometimes called *current flow.)* However, this concept originated prior to the discovery of the electron. Current was then thought to flow from positive (or a higher energy level) to negative (a lower energy level), *but, for our purposes,* current flows from *negative to positive* and consists of the *movement of electrons.* (This concept will be modified when we study semiconductors.)

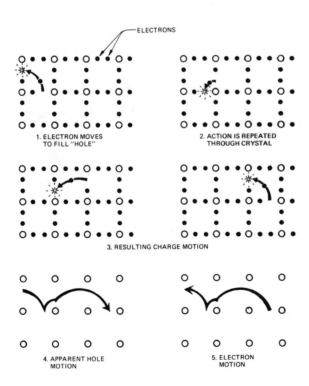

Fig. 2-1: Electron and hole movement

THE SERIES–PARALLEL CONCEPT

A **series circuit** is one in which a number of components are connected in such a way that the *total* current flowing in the circuit passes through each component in completing its path. For example, imagine a lake that is drained by one river which in its course passes through four sets of locks before reaching the sea. All the water leaving the lake passes through these four locks on its way to the sea. This is an example of **series flow**. But suppose someone built a canal by a shorter route and placed four locks in it, then connected the canal to the sea. Now there are two paths by which the lake water can reach the sea; the original course and a parallel course. The waters originate in the same place and end up in the same place but get to their destination by different routes. This is **parallel flow**.

The concept of parallel flow will arise in the examination of many circuit diagrams so it is important to obtain a firm understanding of it now. If in the future you have trouble understanding current and voltage relationships in such circuits, try, if at all possible, to design an analogy using a water flow system—you will find that the two systems function similarly.

VOLTAGE DROP AND RULES FOR SERIES CIRCUITS

At this point it is advantageous to develop the term **voltage drop.** The circuit in Figure 2-2 shows five components (the symbol —◊◊◊◊— means *resistance*) offering opposition to current flow,

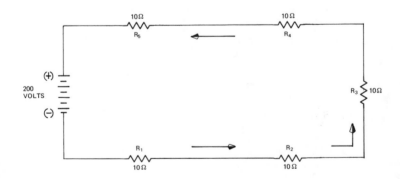

Fig. 2-2: A resistive, series, D.C. circuit

connected in such a way that *all* the current in the circuit passes through each resistance in turn. The electrical pressure producing the current flow is 200 volts provided by a battery. *All* the current flows through each resistor in turn in the same way that water entering a pipeline at one end must pass through each section of pipe before leaving the line at the other end. The total current flow in the circuit shown can therefore be found by using Ohm's Law, which states:

TOTAL CURRENT (I_t) EQUALS TOTAL VOLTAGE (E_t) DIVIDED BY TOTAL RESISTANCE (R_t), OR $I_t = E_t/R_t$.

We have been given the total applied voltage as *200V*. The total resistance can easily be found; since the current flows through one resistor after another the total resistance (as seen by the current) is nothing more than the sum of the individual resistances. This is the first rule of series circuits.

THE TOTAL RESISTANCE IN A SERIES CIRCUIT IS EQUAL TO THE SUM OF THE INDIVIDUAL RESISTANCES OR, $R_t = R_1 + R_2 + R_3 \ldots$ etc.

In the given circuit, $R_t = 50\Omega$. Now that we have both E_t and R_t, we can calculate $I_t = 200 \div 50 = 4$; therefore, $I_t = 4$ amps.

We have now seen that 200 volts of electrical pressure is required to produce a current flow of 4 amps through a resistance of 50 ohms. How would we go about determining the amount of voltage necessary to produce 4 amps of current through *one* of the individual resistances in the circuit? By Ohm's Law, of course: $E = IR$. Choosing R_1, the resistance of $R_1 = 10\Omega$; the current we know is 4 amps; therefore, $E = 4 \times 10 = 40$ volts.

If we used a voltmeter to measure across R_1 we would measure 40 volts; if we measured across all the other resistances together we would measure 160 volts. Therefore, we can say that R_1 has "dropped" 40 volts—or that a "voltage drop" of 40 volts exists across R_1. We can now define **voltage drop** as *the potential required to produce a particular current flow through a portion of a circuit under consideration.*

Since the other resistances in the circuit are also equal to 10Ω each, then each should drop 40 volts. By totalling the drop across each resistor we arrive at 5 x 40 = 200 volts—the total applied voltage.

From this examination we can arrive at another rule of series circuits.

> **IN A SERIES CIRCUIT THE SUM OF THE INDIVIDUAL VOLTAGE DROPS IS EQUAL TO THE APPLIED VOLTAGE, OR,**
> $E_t = E_1 + E_2 + E_3 \ldots$ etc.

The final rule (which we have used but not stated) is:

> **IN A SERIES CIRCUIT, THE CURRENT IS THE SAME AT ALL POINTS IN THE CIRCUIT OR** $I_t = I_1 = I_2 = I_3 \ldots$ etc.

In other words, the current through R_1 is the *same* as the current through R_2, and so forth.

These three rules are invaluable and should be firmly committed to memory.

PARALLEL CIRCUITS

We can now develop the laws governing the distribution of current and voltage in a parallel circuit.

In Figure 2-3, we see that total current flows through R_1 and R_4—but not through R_2 or R_3. At point A, the current is divided, a portion flowing through R_2 and the remainder through R_3. At point B, the two partial currents join and the total current flows again. From this illustration, we can state the rule for current in parallel circuits.

THE TOTAL CURRENT IN A PARALLEL CIRCUIT IS EQUAL TO THE SUM OF THE CURRENTS IN THE INDIVIDUAL BRANCHES.

Stated in another way, $I_t = I_1 + I_2 + I_3$ ... etc. Imagine the water pipe system: total volume flows through R_1 and R_4, but only partial volume flows through each of R_2 and R_3.

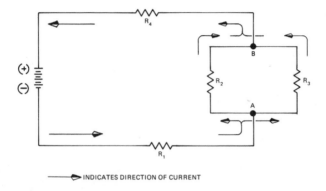

INDICATES DIRECTION OF CURRENT

Fig. 2-3: A series-parallel circuit

A general rule of thumb to remember is that *current takes the path of least resistance*. This means that if a current is faced with two alternate paths, one being a dead short (no resistance) and the other a large resistance, all the current will flow through the short. We can use this rule in cases in which we do not know definite values of resistance and we are required to calculate circuit values.

Example: Two resistors are in parallel, and No. 1 is larger than No. 2. Also, the two values of current flow are 1 amp and 2 amps. Finally, the voltage across both resistors is 10 volts. What is the resistance of R_1? Following the rule, we can conclude that R_1, being the larger, passes the least current. Therefore, the current through R_1 is 1 amp. Since we also know that 10 volts is impressed across the resistor we can easily calculate the resistance by using the formula $R = E/I$, which gives $R = 10/1 = 10$ ohms.

In the previous example we said that the two resistors in parallel had the same voltage across them. Let's see why.

If a difference in energy or pressure exists between two points, and a certain flow rate is obtained between them, the addition of another path for flow between the two points does not affect the pressure difference—but it does affect the overall flow rate.

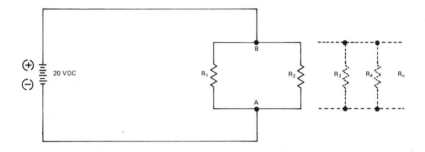

Fig. 2-4: Adding resistances (alternate current paths) in parallel

Therefore, from point A to point B in Figure 2-4, the electrical pressure seen by both legs $(R_1$ and $R_2)$ is the same (20 volts—the potential of the battery). If a third leg were added it also would see the same pressure or voltage). This addition of parallel paths could go on indefinitely—the only thing that would change would be the current through each leg, not the voltage across them. We can now state the rule for voltage in a parallel circuit.

IN A PARALLEL CIRCUIT THE VOLTAGE ACROSS EACH LEG OR BRANCH IS THE SAME.

When dealing with resistances in parallel, we do not calculate an absolute value, rather we calculate what is called the **effective resistance**. For example, the simplest circuit is one in which *equal* resistors are in parallel. In this case the effective resistance is the *resistance of one resistor divided by the number of resistors.*

Example: Two (2) 10 ohm resistors have an effective R of $10 \div 2 = 5$ ohms; or three (3) 12 ohm resistors have an effective R of $12 \div 3 = 4$ ohms.

When resistances are added in parallel, the effective resistance decreases. Why? The explanation is simple. When another path for current flow is added between two points, the net number of free electrons available to carry current increases. From the point of view of total current, what has happened to the circuit resistance? If current carrying ability has increased, then relative opposition (resistance) has decreased.

If resistances are added in parallel, the resultant effective resistance is always *less than or equal to the value of the smallest resistance.*

With unequal resistances in parallel we must use other means to calculate the effective value. In the case of *two* unequal resistances we use the *products over sum* method:

$$R_E = (R_1 \times R_2) \div (R_1 + R_2)$$

Example: If a 12 ohm and a 4 ohm resistance are in parallel, R_E is: $(12 \times 4) \div (12 + 4) = 48/16 = 3$ ohms.

When we have more than two unequal resistances in parallel, two can be calculated at one time; their effective value is then used in parallel with the next, and so on, or we can use the following reciprocal method.

THE EFFECTIVE RESISTANCE OF PARALLEL RESISTANCES IS EQUAL TO THE RECIPROCAL OF THE SUM OF THE RECIPROCALS OF THE INDIVIDUAL RESISTANCES.

$$R_E = \frac{1}{\dfrac{1}{R_1} + \dfrac{1}{R_2} + \dfrac{1}{R_3} + \ldots \text{etc.}}$$

In discussing the types of circuits we have covered so far you should always remember to be concerned with:

1. The total voltage and the drops across each part of the circuit.
2. The total current and the current in each part of the circuit.
3. The total resistance, effective resistances, and the resistance of each part of the circuit.

SERIES-PARALLEL CIRCUITS

The circuit shown in Figure 2-3 is a series-parallel one. We have discussed only the parallel portion, however. In examining series-parallel circuits all the rules we have examined up to this point are employed. It is easier if the circuit is reduced step by step to an equivalent circuit (which can be done to any circuit). Look at the circuit shown in· Figure 2-5A. At first glance it may seem complex, but let us take it down to a simple series equivalent circuit in a step-by-step method. It is best to start combining values at a point farthest from the voltage source.

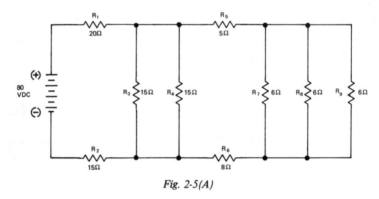

Fig. 2-5(A)

In Figure 2-5A, we first find the equivalent resistance of R_7, R_8 and R_9 by dividing the value of one resistor by the total number of resistances in parallel. (Remember, this method can be used only when the parallel resistances are *equal*). We obtain 6÷3

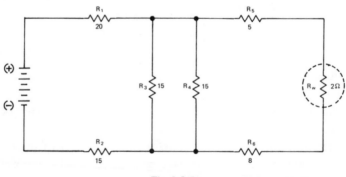

Fig. 2-5(B)

= 2Ω. In Figure 2-5*B*, resistances *7*, *8*, and *9* are replaced by their equivalent, R_W.

The sum of R_5, R_6 and R_W (sum because these three resistances are in series with each other) equals 15. They are now replaced in Figure 2-5*C* by resistor R_X.

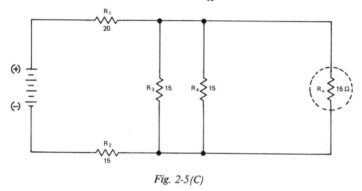

Fig. 2-5(C)

R_X is now seen to be a parallel resistance along with R_3 and R_4. The equivalent resistance of these legs is 15÷3 = 5Ω. This whole segment can be replaced by R_Y = 5Ω, as shown in Figure 2-5*D*.

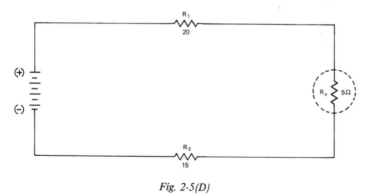

Fig. 2-5(D)

The complex circuit shown in *A* has now been reduced to the simple series circuit shown in *D*. The total resistance of the overall circuit can quickly be found by adding the values of R_1, R_Y and R_2: 20 + 5 + 15 = 40Ω. The final circuit shown in Figure 2-5*E* shows R_Z representing the overall effective resistance of the circuit. The total current can now be calculated using Ohm's Law—$I = E \div R$, or $I = 80 \div 40 = 2$ amps.

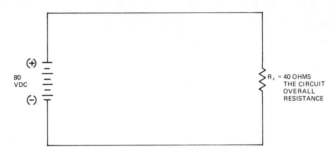

Fig. 2-5(E)

THE WHEATSTONE BRIDGE

The Wheatstone bridge is a relatively simple device used in many analytical instruments from flame photometers to gas chromatographs. Its theory of operation makes use of the laws of parallel circuits previously mentioned. A typical Wheatstone bridge is shown on the left of Fig. 2-6. On the right is the same bridge circuit drawn in a simplified manner.

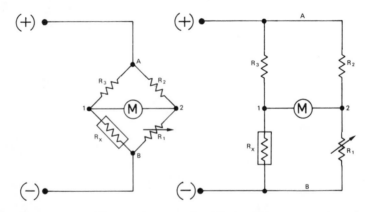

Fig. 2-6: Two forms of a Wheatstone bridge

In the sample circuit shown, R_X is the **test** or unknown resistance. R_1 is a variable or **reference resistance**. The bridge is "balanced" when the ratios R_3/R_X and R_2/R_1 are equal. When the balanced condition exists, the voltage dropped across R_X equals the voltage across R_1. In this case, the potential at point 1 is the same as the potential at point 2. You will observe that a galvanometer (M) is hooked between points 1 and 2. With no difference in potential across it, no current flows through the galvanometer, and there is no deflection of its pointer. This shows the bridge is balanced.

The resistor R_X can be of many types; often it is a semiconductor. It may be a photoconductive cell, made of material which changes its ability to conduct current when light strikes it. Other types of sensing devices may be used to convert other kinds of energy changes in a test system to equivalent changes in their own values of resistance. Once R_X changes value, the bridge becomes unbalanced. For example, if R_X increases, the voltage drop across it increases. This makes point 1 positive with respect to point 2. The difference in potential across the galvanometer causes a current to flow and the galvanometer needle to deflect. Balance may be restored by an adjustment of R_1. The amount of galvanometer deflection is proportional to the change in R_X.

The Wheatstone bridge circuit is used in many analytical instruments. Through various electrical and electromechanical methods, this type of circuit may be used to control a strip chart recorder, meter, or digital read-out device. Remembering that the Wheatstone bridge is a simple parallel circuit will help to make understanding such devices a little easier.

CIRCUIT LOADING AND IMPEDANCE

When considering parallel circuits it is also convenient to introduce the concepts of **loading** and **impedance**. From a simplified point of view, the analysis of circuits reveals that any electrical circuit can be considered as functioning in one or more of the following ways:

1. As a *power source,* driving one or more other circuits;
2. As a *signal source,* yielding information (a voltage) that is fed into another circuit;
3. As a *load,* taking information (a voltage) from a source and modifying it in some way. (Often a circuit acts both as a load

for a circuit that precedes it and as a source for another circuit that follows it.)

To understand circuit loading, we must briefly consider the meaning of *impedance*. Impedance will be more fully explained in later chapters but, for the present, we may think of it as follows.

Resistance, we have seen, is one kind of opposition to current flow. Resistance is important in both direct and alternating current circuits. In alternating current circuits, another kind of current-opposing effect called **reactance** is caused by the presence of capacitors and inductors (both of which will be discussed later). The combined current-opposing effect of reactance and resistance is called **impedance** (symbol Z; units, ohms).

Resistance has a fixed or manually variable magnitude that is independent of the applied signal's frequency. Impedance, on the other hand, is a dynamic effect whose magnitude is frequency-dependent. When an AC circuit is to be analyzed, the values of impedance shown by its different ends (input and output) become important factors in its evaluation.

In evaluating the operation of a particular circuit, we look on whatever comes before it as the **source** and whatever comes after it as its **load.** We then work from the source, through the circuit under examination, to its load—considering all the possible impedances, as follows:

1. Impedance of the signal source as seen by* the circuit.
2. Input impedance of the circuit as seen by the source.
3. Output impedance of the circuit as seen by the load.
4. Load impedance as seen by the circuit.

A simplified diagram showing these impedances is given in Figure 2-7. Note that *1* and *2* form a parallel circuit as do *3* and *4*. These two pairs of impedances are important in connection with loading. Figure 2-8 is an example of this.

Let us assume there exists a signal source with impedance R of 10Ω and a current of 10 milliamps. The signal voltage developed by the source is 100 millivolts. If we attach a load (voltmeter) having an impedance of 100Ω, the load forms a parallel path for source current. By drawing some of the source current, the load

---

*The phrase "as seen by" means the value that would be measured by an appropriate ohmmeter replacing the circuit that is "seeing."

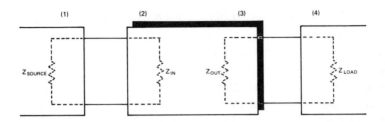

Fig. 2-7: Relative circuit impedances

causes the voltage drop across R to become less than 100 mv—and the voltmeter will indicate an inaccurate value. In order *not* to load the source, the ideal voltmeter should have a high input impedance (at least one hundred times that of the source) and draw virtually *no* current.

From this example we can conclude that, to prevent reduction of voltage due to loading, one of the two following circuit conditions must be satisfied:

1. The load must have a high input impedance and therefore draw virtually no current;

2. The source must be able to compensate for any load current variations without a change in its output voltage.

The example in the previous paragraph required the first

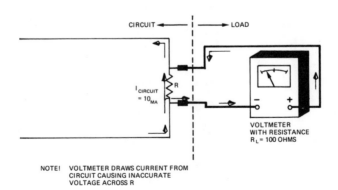

Fig. 2-8: Voltmeter loading a circuit

condition. An example of the second condition is found in a regulated power supply.

Let us assume that a power supply is set for a required output voltage *without* a load. As soon as the load is connected, it provides a parallel current path along with the power supply, draws current, and consequently results in a lower supplied voltage than originally set, unless the power supply is "regulated" in such a way as to hold the voltage constant.

In the case of a load whose current requirements constantly change, the result would be a constantly changing supply voltage unless the power supply could compensate for the changes. This problem will be considered in more detail in the discussion of power supplies.

The fundamental point to keep in mind with respect to DC circuit loading is that any time a parallel resistance is added to a circuit, unless its value is at least one hundred times that of the circuit, it will draw enough current to cause a significant change in the circuit voltage. Due to the additional fact that reactances are frequency-dependent, when loading occurs in AC circuits, not only voltage attenuation can result, but also signal distortion.

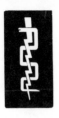# basic electromagnetism

CHAPTER 3

MAGNETISM

Due to the condensed and descriptive nature of this volume, some information pertaining to magnets will not be covered. We will, however, discuss the properties of magnets—but without delving into extensive explanations.

A **magnet** is a material having the ability to attract iron or iron alloys. There are *natural* and *artificial* magnets.

A natural magnet is a form of iron ore called *magnetite* (or lodestone) possessing magnetic qualities in its unrefined state.

An artificial magnet is produced by contact or close approach between a magnetic material and a natural magnet, or by inducing magnetism through electrical means. The magnets produced electrically are stronger and consequently more common than those produced by contact.

Artificial magnets can also be divided into two groups: *permanent* magnets and *temporary* magnets. Temporary magnets lose their magnetic quality soon after the magnetizing force has been removed and are used in relays, circuit-breakers, and switches. Permanent magnets are able to retain their magnetic qualities for a relatively long period of time after removal of the magnetizing force and find use in the movements of galvanometers and other meters.

The region around a magnet, where its influence can be felt, is termed its **magnetic field**. The effects of this field are not evenly distributed, but instead are stronger near the ends and weaker toward the center. The stronger regions are the **poles** of the magnet. Figure 3-1 depicts the distribution of the field around a bar magnet.

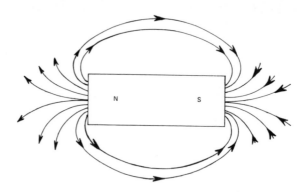

Fig. 3-1: Lines of force around a magnet

Weber's molecular theory of magnetism is the most popular theory in use today, Briefly, it is based on the assumption that all molecules of a magnetic material are individual magnets. In an unmagnetized material molecules are oriented in random fashion, while in a magnetized material molecules are aligned in a definite direction. As the strength of the magnetizing force is increased, more "molecular magnets" align themselves until all are aligned in the same direction—the material is then *saturated* (Figure 3-2).

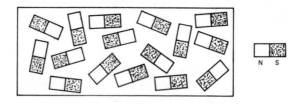

Fig. 3-2(A): Unmagnetized material showing random alignment of molecular magnets

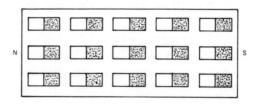

Fig. 3-2(B): Magnetized material showing symmetrical alignment of molecular magnets

The following list is a summary of some of the interesting properties of the invisible force field around a magnet.

1. The force field can be depicted by **lines of force**. Such lines are drawn in the direction of the magnetic force, and the *density* of the lines represents the *strength of the field.*
2. These lines form closed loops travelling north to south *outside* the magnet, south to north *inside* the magnet.
3. Lines of force *never* cross each other.
4. Lines of force expand or contract when a force is exerted upon them and return to their original state when the force is removed (somewhat like rubber bands).
5. No material can completely prevent their passage, but they become more densely packed passing through magnetic materials than through air or nonmagnets.
6. The strength of the force field at any point is measured in lines of force per square centimeter or **flux density**. The unit of flux density is the **gauss** (symbol: B).

ELECTROMAGNETISM

The two invisible forces of electricity and magnetism are virtually inseparable because of their close relationship which was first shown to exist by Hans C. Oersted, a Danish physicist. Oersted found that around a current-carrying conductor there exists a magnetic field aligned in such a way that the field is always tangent to a circle drawn around the conductor. He also found that the strength of the field is: (1) *inversely proportional* to the distance from the conductor, and (2) *directly proportional* to the amount of current flowing through the conductor.

The lines of force around a conductor-carrying current travel in a clockwise or a counterclockwise direction, depending on the direction of current flow and in accordance with the **Left Hand Rule**:

IF YOU GRASP A CONDUCTOR WITH YOUR LEFT HAND WITH THE THUMB POINTING IN THE DIRECTION OF CURRENT FLOW, YOUR FINGERS WILL INDICATE THE DIRECTION OF THE MAGNETIC LINES OF FORCE.

If a straight conductor is bent into a loop, the lines of force will concentrate within the loop because all the lines of force enter the loop from one side. If the wire is formed into a coil, the magnetic fields around each turn will have the same direction and will be concentrated within each loop. Figure 3-3 shows a magnetic field around and within a coil.

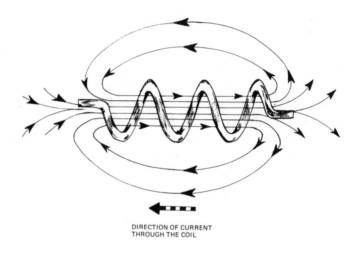

DIRECTION OF CURRENT
THROUGH THE COIL

Fig. 3-3: Magnetic field around a coiled current carrying wire

Electromagnetic Induction

Michael Faraday discovered that a current could be induced into a conductor by a magnetic field, *if there was relative motion between the two.* The operation of electrical generators and motors is based on this principle (termed **electromagnetic induction.** To demonstrate, take a permanent horseshoe magnet and a conductor connected to a galvanometer (a device used to detect very small amounts of current flow); then move the conductor up and down between the poles of the magnet. You will see the galvanometer needle move, indicating a current is flowing in the conductor. You will also find the indicator deflects the greatest amount when the conductor is moved *perpendicular* to the lines of force and not at all when it is moved *parallel* to them.

The amount of current induced is proportional to two factors:
1. Strength of the field (density of lines of force);
2. Speed of the conductor.
One can increase the amount of current induced in any of the following ways.
  1. Increase field strength (flux density) thus increasing the rate at which lines are cut.
  2. Increase the speed of the conductor, which has the same effect.
  3. Increase the number of conductors by forming a coil.
It is important to remember that:

ANY CHANGE OF CURRENT FLOW IN A CONDUCTOR IS ALWAYS ACCOMPANIED BY A CHANGE IN THE MAGNETIC FIELD SURROUNDING THE CONDUCTOR.

An increase in the current causes the field to expand; a decrease allows it to collapse.

We will now develop the principal of **mutual induction**. It has been stated previously that a conductor moved through a magnetic field has a current induced into it. To obtain this induced current, *either* the conductor *or* the magnetic field can be moving. Therefore, if we place a conductor (through which no current is flowing) within an expanding or collapsing field, lines of force are cut and current is induced into the conductor. We can accomplish this if through one coil (called the *primary*) we run an alternating current, which is constantly changing in direction and magnitude. Around this coil a periodically expanding and collapsing magnetic field will be produced. If another coil (called the *secondary*) is placed within the influence of the magnetic field of the primary coil, a current will be induced into the secondary coil. The action or principle by which this is accomplished is known as **mutual induction**. The resulting device is called a *transformer*. Another principle known as *self-induction* will be discussed later.

Generators and Motors

Every generator or motor consists basically of the two functional parts mentioned in the previous paragraph, a conductor and a magnetic field.

The interaction between a magnetic field and a conductor works in either of two ways:

1. A varying current through a conductor causes a varying magnetic field around the conductor. This field interacts with a stationary magnetic field, the result being movement of the conductor. (It is this principle upon which motors operate.) Most laboratory centrifuges function this way, using a motor to turn the centrifuge head.

2. A conductor caused to move through a magnetic field by mechanical action will have a current flow induced into it due to the conductor cutting magnetic lines of force. This is the principle upon which generators function. A generator in which a permanent magnet provides the magnetic field is called a **magneto**; if the field is produced by an electro-magnet, it is called a **dynamo**. The part of the machine which contains the conductors is the **armature**.

A **generator** is a device (**magneto** or **dynamo**) which *changes mechanical energy into electrical energy.* Let's see how!

A conductor shaped as shown in Figure 3-4 is made to rotate in a magnetic field.

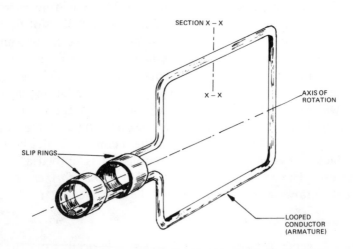

Fig. 3-4: Armature and slip rings of an AC generator (highly simplified)

Relating the cross sections X-X in Figure 3-4 to Figure 3-6*B*, the operation of a generator can be analyzed. Each small circle represents the *same conductor segment* in one position after another as it moves clockwise, first down and then up through the magnetic field. At *A,* the conductor is travelling parallel to the flux lines—no lines are cut, no current is induced. As soon as the conductor begins to cut the magnetic lines of force by moving down, a current is induced into it such that it flows into the page. This can easily be seen by applying the left-hand rule. The conductor would tend to distort the lines of force as indicated in Figure 3-5.

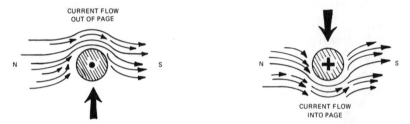

Fig. 3-5: A conductor moving through a magnetic field

Applying the left-hand rule to Figure 3-5, we find that the current induced flows into the page when the conductor is moving down and the current flows out of the page when the conductor moves up. Referring back to Figure 3-6*B*, we see that:

From *A* to *C:* The rate of cutting lines gradually increases until *C* when a maximum is reached. The induced current increases proportionately to a maximum at *C.*

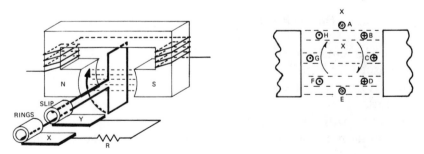

Figures 3-6(A), and (B):   Adapted from Air Force manual 52-8, electronic circuit analysis – modified by the author – courtesy of the United States Air Force

From *C* to *E*: The rate of cutting lines decreases until *E*, where no lines are being cut. The current induced decreases proportionately to zero at *E*.

From *E* to *G*: The conductor is now moving up. The induced current is now in the opposite direction. The number of lines cut per unit time gradually increases until *G* when the maximum is reached. The current increases from zero to a maximum at *G*.

From *G* to *A*: The number of lines cut per unit time gradually decreases—the current induced decreases proportionately to zero at *A* once again.

As can be seen from a diagram (Figure 3-6*C*) of the induced current, the output from this device is alternating current. The induced current is picked off the conductor by *slip rings*. Analyzing Figure 3-6*A*, we see that the current through *R* alternates in direction—consequently, we call the device an **alternating current generator.**

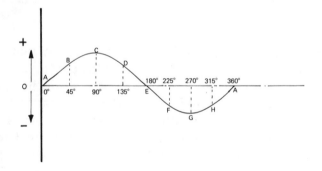

Fig. 3-6(C):   Wave form of magnetically induced current

Fundamentally a DC generator differs from an AC generator in one aspect only. Instead of using simple slip rings to pick off the current flow, a device known as a **commutator** is used.

Notice that with an AC generator, each slip ring is in contact at all times with its own brush. In a simple DC generator the commutator functions at two half rings each insulated from the other.

Figure 3-7 *A* shows the operation of a simple DC generator. In *A*, C_1 is moving up and current is induced in the direction

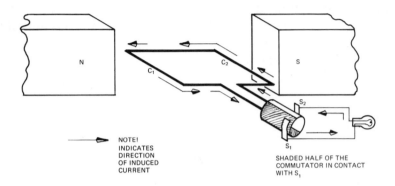

Fig. 3-7(A):   Simplified DC generator

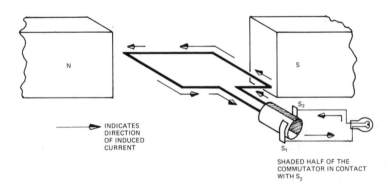

Fig. 3-7(B):

shown, flowing onto the shaded part of the commutator B_1. It is then picked up by brush S_1 and passes through the lamp, back to S_2, on to the unshaded part of the commutator and back into the loop through C_2. As the loop reaches the vertical position, no current is induced and the brushes touch insulating material between the two parts of the commutator. In B, a half cycle later, C_1 is moving down, current is induced back out through C_2, on to the unshaded part of the commutator, is picked up by brush S_1, passes through the lamp to S_2, passes through the shaded part of the commutator, and goes back into the loop through C_1. Since the direction of current flow through the lamp is always the same, we have a DC output. By employing more than one conductor, we can obtain a more even output, since at any one instant one conductor will be cutting maximum lines of force and, therefore, will be carrying a maximum current.

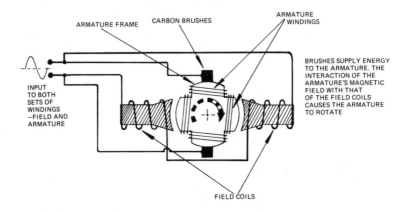

Fig. 3-8: Pictorial diagram of a simple motor

We have seen that mechanical energy rotating a conductor in a magnetic field generates electricity. Employing the reverse sequence, we can cause electrical energy to rotate a conductor, thereby producing mechanical energy. This is done in an **electric motor.** A number of electromagnetic fields are produced on an *armature capable of rotating.* At the same time, electromagnetic fields are produced by two stationary *field coils.* These coils are placed so that the armature is between them. The multiple armature fields, attempting to align themselves with the stationary fields, cause the armature to rotate. Figure 3-8 shows the relationship of the field coils to the armature.

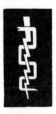 types of meter movements

CHAPTER 4

Diagnostic instruments found in today's clinical laboratories and hospitals for the most part employ meters as read-out or monitoring devices. Although the meters and the instruments of which they are part serve in various measuring capacities, from indirectly reflecting changes in light intensity to changes in pH, they all function in a similar manner. A change in the parameter under analysis produces an electrical change, which, in turn, causes movement of a meter needle. Today, many instruments are appearing with digital (numerical) read-out systems. However, since meters are not currently in danger of becoming obsolete it will be to our advantage to understand something about them.

A meter consists of three basic parts: the *movement,* the *face* (or scale), and the *case.* The meter case and scale vary with the purpose of each meter, but all movements function by applications of either electromagnetic or electrostatic theory.

Most meters employ applications of electromagnetic theory. A current-carrying conductor is placed within the field of a permanent magnet. When current flows through the conductor it produces its own magnetic field. The second field interacts with the stationary one, thereby causing the conductor to move. This operating principle is the basis on which all D'Arsonval or moving coil movements function.

There are three other types of meter movements in use today:

1. The moving iron vane movement;
2. The electrostatic movement;
3. The dynamometer movement.

Of the four types, the D'Arsonval is the most widely used. We will examine the D'Arsonval and the moving iron vane movements in some detail; the electrostatic and dynamometer movements are not commonly found in clinical instruments.

THE D'ARSONVAL GALVANOMETER

The D'Arsonval meter movement is a modification of the original D'Arsonval galvanometer. (A **galvanometer** is a device for detecting minute amounts of current flow). Consequently, it is only natural that we first examine the operating principles of the galvanometer. Its basic parts are:

1. A permanent magnet;
2. A moving element, consisting of a plastic support bobbin around which is wound a current-carrying coil; a small reflecting mirror is also mounted upon the bobbin;
3. A highly flexible current-carrying spiral spring.

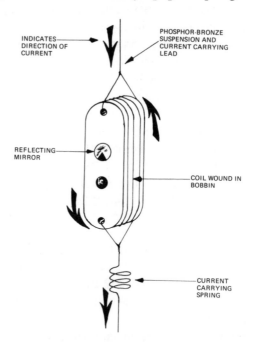

INDICATES
DIRECTION OF
CURRENT

PHOSPHOR-BRONZE
SUSPENSION AND
CURRENT CARRYING
LEAD

REFLECTING
MIRROR

COIL WOUND IN
BOBBIN

CURRENT
CARRYING
SPRING

Fig. 4-1: *D'Arsonval string galvanometer bobbin assembly (courtesy Philco-Ford Corp., Tech-Rep Division, Fort Washington, Penna.)*

Figure 4-1 illustrates the moving element and the spiral spring. The bobbin is suspended by a phosphor bronze current-carrying wire, which, in turn is wound around the bobbin and then attached to the spring. The path of the detected current is through the suspension wire, around the coil, and through the spring.

The device operates as follows:

a. The detected current flows through the wire, coil, and spring. A magnetic field is generated around the bobbin.

b. The generated field attempts to align itself with the permanent field. The torque produced by this interaction causes the bobbin to turn.

c. A light beam shines on the mirror. When the bobbin moves, the mirror moves, and the direction of the *reflected* light beam changes.

d. When the current ceases to flow through the coil, its magnetic field degenerates. The spring below the bobbin returns the bobbin to its original, or zero, position.

With no current flowing, the reflected image is mechanically adjusted to center scale; current flow in either direction through the coil (positive or negative) may then be detected. The image will be moved to the right for current flow in one direction and to the left for current flow in the opposite direction.

The galvanometer just described is a very sensitive instrument since only a small magnetic force is needed to overcome the inertia of the suspended bobbin.

THE D'ARSONVAL METER MOVEMENT

As noted previously, the D'Arsonval meter movement (Figure 4-2A) is a modified galvanometer. It is not as sensitive as the galvanometer just described since more energy is required to overcome the inertia of the moving element.

The movement consists of:

1. A permanent magnet;
2. A moving element, wire wound, with an attached indicator needle;
3. Jeweled bearings;
4. A moving element mounting;
5. Springs (controlling elements).

The movement employs the same operating principle as the galvanometer. The magnetic field produced by the coil attempts to align itself with the fixed field; the amount of deflection from the

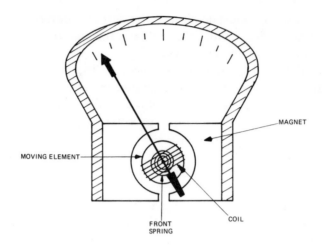

Fig. 4-2(A): Typical meter movement

zero position is proportional to the current flowing through the coil.

In Figure 4-2*B*, the poles of the permanent magnet are curved around the moving element. This insures right-angle orientation between the opposing fields, resulting in accurate proportionality between the current and displacement of the meter movement. This design feature allows use of a *linear* meter scale rather than a nonlinear or quadratic scale.

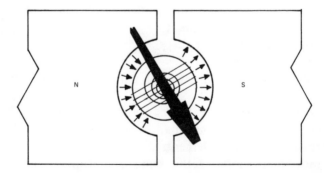

Fig. 4-2(B): Curved poles allow right angle orientation of magnetic field (courtesy Philco-Ford Corp., Tech-Rep Division, Fort Washington, Penna.)

Dual opposing springs are used with this movement to eliminate any deflection caused by temperature effects upon the springs. With one spring, a temperature change may cause contraction or expansion of the spring, thereby pulling the movement in one direction. With an opposing spring added, any temperature change is reflected in both springs, and the two springs are so arranged that the pull of one is nullified by the equal and opposite pull of the other. In addition, the springs act as a controlling element in that they provide an opposing force against up-scale pointer movement. As the pointer moves farther up-scale, the opposing force increases. The pointer stops at the correct point on the scale when the deflecting force equals the opposing force of the springs.

The pointer is balanced by placing three spring balance weights on arms around the pivot point. These weights and the jeweled bearings in which the moving element are mounted are prone to shock damage which can result in the movement being inaccurate.

THE IRON VANE MOVEMENT

The iron vane movement consists of a coil and two easily magnetized iron vanes, one fixed and one movable. An indicating pointer is attached to the movable vane, while a retaining spring keeps the vanes adjacent to each other when no current is flowing through the coil. When current flows through the coil, a magnetic field is produced and magnetizes both vanes. The lines of force pass in the same direction through both vanes; therefore, the vanes are magnetized so that the poles are aligned, north-to-north and south-to-south. Since like poles repel, the movable vane is deflected away from the stationary vane.

The magnetic polarity of the vanes is dependent upon the direction of current flow through the coil, but both vanes are affected the same so that, even if the direction of the current flow in the coil is reversed, the magnetic poles will still repel each other. Consequently, an iron vane movement can detect direct or alternating current without further modification.

It is important to know that iron vane movements cause pointer deflection in an amount proportional to the square of the current flow, rather than in direct proportion (as in the case of the D'Arsonval linear movement). For example, if current through a coil doubles, the field around *each* vane will be twice as strong; the combined repulsion of the two vanes will be four times as great, resulting in a pointer deflection four times as great. For this reason moving vane meters employ nonlinear "quadratic" or "square law" scales.

DAMPING

A difficulty common to all meter movement is pointer oscillation; the pointer tends to overshoot the true reading and then oscillate about it, finally coming to rest. The oscillations are the result of tension in the spiral springs opposing the motion of the meter movement, and inertia of the moving element. Damping of unwanted oscillations can be brought about by electromagnetic or mechanical action.

Electromagnetic damping is obtained by winding the meter coil on an aluminum frame suspended within the field of the permanent magnet. Movement of the frame will induce "eddy" currents within the frame. These currents produce a magnetic field of their own, which tends to oppose the motion of the coil. Aluminum is difficult to magnetize; consequently, the strength of the "frame field" is only enough to place a small drag on the coil's motion, thereby reducing small rapid oscillations, but not hampering the slower up scale movement of the pointer. The strength of the induced field can limit oscillation—not movement produced by the coil.

Mechanical damping is obtained by connecting a flat vane to the pointer. The vane is then placed within a semi-airtight chamber. As the element and pointer move, air is compressed on one side of the vane opposing any rapid swing of the device. The vane allows air to pass around it, so slow movement is not hampered, while the tendency for overshooting the actual stop point is reduced.

A combination of both types of damping may be used in some applications.

SENSITIVITY

The sensitivity of meter movement depends upon the amount of current in milliamps necessary to operate the moving elements of the meter. The movement requiring the least amount of current for full scale deflection is considered to be the most sensitive. The amount of current required is in turn dependent upon the number of turns of wire in the moving coil, as well as the inertia that must be overcome to produce movement, the friction of the bearings, characteristics of the springs, and other factors. (Therefore, a galvanometer such as the one previously described would be more sensitive than the D'Arsonval movement mentioned due to its having less inertia.) The larger the coil of a movement (*i.e.,* more turns), the stronger the magnetic field produced, and consequently, the less current required to cause full scale deflection.

Since all substances have some electrical resistance, the moving coil also exhibits resistance, known as **internal meter resistance.** Internal meter resistance is that resistance (of the coil itself) which must be overcome by the current flowing through the movement. With this in mind, it is obvious that a small voltage is dropped across meter movements. Therefore, although sensitivity is defined as the amount of current required to produce full scale deflection, it is also related to internal meter resistance and meter voltage drop (when full scale deflection current is flowing). Meter resistance (symbol, R_m) is expressed in ohms; full scale voltage is usually expressed in millivolts. Full scale current can be expressed in microamps, milliamps, or amps, relative to the use of the instrument.

Example: A movement whose R_m = 50 ohms and which requires 1 ma of current for full scale deflection has a sensitivity of 1 ma and its full scale voltage ($E = I \times R$) is 1 × 50 = 50 millivolts.

Meter sensitivity is also described by the term *ohms per volt,* which is the internal meter resistance divided by the full scale voltage. More sensitive meters have higher ohms-per-volt ratios.

EXTENDING METER RANGE

We have just seen such an example of a meter movement with a sensitivity of 1 ma and R_m of 50Ω. Such a movement alone would be of limited use. The maximum current it could detect or measure would be 1 milliamp; the largest voltage, 50 millivolts. To measure 50 milliamps or 500 volts, we must extend the meter's range. We do this in two ways, depending on whether the meter is being used to measure current or voltage.

Extending the Range of an Ammeter

The following example shows us how this is accomplished (Figure 4-3).

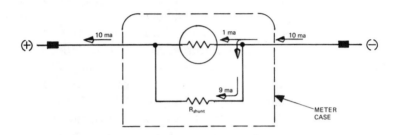

Fig. 4-3: Extending the range of an ammeter (see text)

Example: Let us assume that a 50 mv, 0-1 ma meter is available and it must be used to measure a maximum of 10 ma. We can do this in two ways:

1. First, we determine $R_m \cdot R_m = E_{fs}/I_{fs}$. where R_m = meter resistance in ohms; E_{fs} = full scale volts in mv; and I_{fs} = full scale current in ma. In this case $R_m = 50/1 = 50$ ohms.

2. Since only 1 ma can flow through the movement, 9 ma must be "shunted" around the movement. To accomplish this, a resistor is placed in parallel with the movement. Of the 10 ma of maximum possible circuit current, 1 ma flows through the meter and 9 ma through the "shunt" resistance. Since R_s (shunt resistance) is in parallel with R_m, both will feel the same voltage drop. Therefore, it is a simple calculation to determine the value of $R_s \cdot R_s = E_{fs}/I_{R\,s}$ where E_{fs} = full scale voltage (mv), and $I_{R\,s}$ = current through R_s (at full scale). Therefore, R_s = 50 mv/9ma = 5.55 ohms.

This general formula can be used to determine the shunt resistor for any value of current to be measured once meter sensitivities are known.

Shunt resistances are very critical, since a small deviation can cause too much current to flow through the movement.

Extending The Range of A Voltmeter

A meter movement measuring current flow also has a voltage drop across it. If it became necessary to measure voltages up to 10 volts, and the only meter available was the one used in the previous paragraph, how could this be accomplished? The solution is relatively simple. Since the maximum value to be measured is 10 volts and the meter can tolerate a maximum of 50 mv, then 9.950 volts must be dropped across another resistance. This is done by placing a resistance *in series* with the meter (Figure 4-4). The resistor is known as the "multiplier," designated R_x. The value of R_x can be computed by dividing the voltage range required by the full scale current and subtracting R_m from the result. The answer gives R_x.

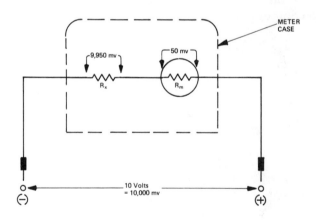

Fig. 4-4: Extending the range of a voltmeter (see text)

Example: For a 50 mv, 0-1 ma movement, the multiplier for a 10 volt range is $10/1 \times 10^{-3} = 10,000\Omega$, $R_m = 50/1 = 50\Omega$, $R_x = 10,000 - 50 = 9950$ ohms.

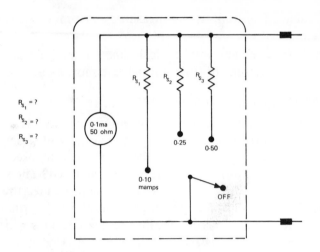

Fig. 4-5(A): A simplified multiple range ammeter

Figure 4-5 shows the schematic diagrams for (*A*) an ammeter with three ranges, and (*B*) a voltmeter with three ranges. (See if you can compute the proper R_s and R_x values.)

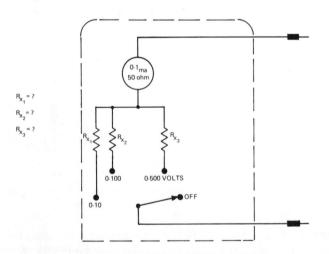

Fig. 4-5(B): A simplified multiple range voltmeter

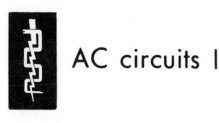

AC circuits I

CHAPTER 5

TERMINOLOGY

Before attempting to study AC circuits and associated components, the general terminology and definitions used with AC waveforms should first be examined.

As previously stated, alternating current periodically changes direction. The wave pattern is repeated over and over again. A single cycle represents one of these repetitions. Figure 5-1*A* represents two cycles of a sinusoidal alternating current (or voltage). Point *A* to point *B* represents one full period or cycle of the waveform. There are 360 electrical degrees in a cycle. Points 1, 2, 3, and 4 are 90, 180, 270, and 360 degrees respectively, from point *A*.

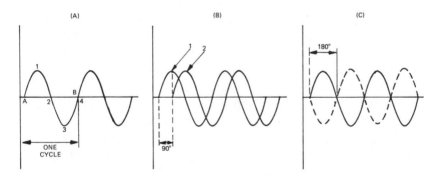

Fig. 5-1: AC waveforms – terminology (see text)

Frequency refers to the number of cycles of a particular waveform that are generated per second. If the signal in Figure 5-1*A* represented a 60 cps signal, it would mean that the signal was being generated 60 times per second. (The term *cycles per second*

49

—cps—is no longer used. Instead 60 cps is given as 60Hz—**hertz** being the new unit of frequency.) In such a case, the time for one cycle, or the **period,** would be 1/60th of a second. The relationship between period (time for one cycle) and the frequency of the signal is a reciprocal one for T = 1/F and F = 1/T (where *T* and *F* refer to period and frequency, respectively.)

Using one signal as a reference, we can determine the time relationship (or **phase difference**) between that signal and one or more other waveforms. Figure 5-1*B* shows an example of two waveforms 90° out of phase. Waveform No. 1 is at its maximum positive swing at the time waveform No. 2 is beginning its positive swing. Figure 5-1*C* represents two waveforms 180° out of phase. If two such voltages are injected into a circuit, both of equal magnitude, the resultant, or net, voltage felt by the circuit will be zero, since one signal cancels the other.

By the use of components called **reactors,** selected phase changes can be developed that enable the engineer to mold waveforms that can be combined to give desired shapes and sizes necessary for special functions in electronic circuitry.

IMPEDANCE AND REACTORS

In DC circuits, resistance is regarded as the only opposition to current flow. In AC circuits, however, another type of opposition to current flow appears. Whereas resistance is a static entity (its value remains the same regardless of changes in frequency, voltage, or phase of the applied signal), this AC circuit phenomenon is a dynamic entity; its value varies relative to the frequency of the applied signal. Such opposition is termed **reactance.** The symbol for reactance is X and it is measured in ohms. In a DC circuit, resistance alone provides the major opposition to current. In an AC circuit, resistance becomes a part of the overall opposition since there is opposition offered also by the reactive components. The total opposition to current flow in an AC circuit is a function of resistance and reactance, collectively termed **impedance** and given the symbol $Z,$ also measured in ohms.

The two components supplying reactance to an AC circuit are **inductors** and **capacitors.** These devices are referred to as **reactors,** because they do not *dissipate* electrical energy in the form of heat (as do resistors) but alternately *store* energy and then deliver it back to the circuit. Inductors store energy in an electromagnetic field; capacitors store energy in an electrostatic field. Time is required to accumulate, store, and then release energy; this should be a clue to the fact that reactors produce changes in phase relationships.

INDUCTORS

Electromagnetic theory (discussed in Chapter 3) tells us that, when current flows through a conductor, a magnetic field is generated around the conductor. If such a conductor is shaped to form a coil, the magnetic field generated is aligned so that the individual field segments produced around each turn of the coil combine, resulting in an intensification of the field strength within the inner portion (or core) of the coil (*cf* Chapter 3, Figure 3-3). One end of the coil becomes the north pole and the other the south pole. It is in such a way that coils or inductors store electrical energy. The ability to store energy in an electromagnetic field makes inductors infinitely useful in electronics.

INDUCTANCE AND BACK EMF

If the current through a conductor is a direct current, the magnetic field around the conductor will be stationary, with no variation in size or intensity (Figure 5-2). When an alternating

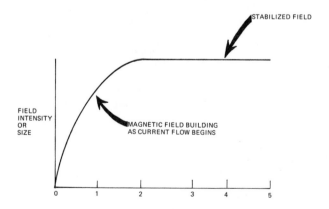

Fig. 5-2: Graph of magnetic field around a conductor passing a D.C. current

current is passed through an inductor, the magnetic field produced varies at the same rate and in proportion to the magnitude of the current. The result is a constantly moving magnetic field. This moving magnetic field, upon cutting the adjacent turns of the coil, produces what is known as back or *counter-EMF*. Let us see how this occurs.

As the current begins to increase through the coil the magnetic lines of flux around each individual turn of the coil expand. The expanding field cuts through the adjacent turns of the coil (Figure 5-3).

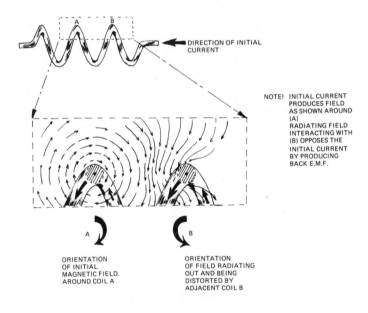

DIRECTION OF INITIAL CURRENT

NOTE! INITIAL CURRENT PRODUCES FIELD AS SHOWN AROUND (A) RADIATING FIELD INTERACTING WITH (B) OPPOSES THE INITIAL CURRENT BY PRODUCING BACK E.M.F.

ORIENTATION OF INITIAL MAGNETIC FIELD. AROUND COIL A

ORIENTATION OF FIELD RADIATING OUT AND BEING DISTORTED BY ADJACENT COIL B

Fig. 5-3: Diagram of self inductance producing back E.M.F.

NOTE: There is relative motion between the magnetic field and the conductor.

The relative motion between the two results in a current being induced into the adjacent turns such that *it opposes the current flow that originally produced the field.* This phenomenon is known as **Lenz's Law**, which states:

WHEN A CURRENT IS INDUCED IN A COIL AS A RESULT OF ANY VARIATION IN THE MAGNETIC FIELD SURROUNDING THE COIL, THE INDUCED CURRENT IS IN SUCH A DIRECTION AS TO OPPOSE THE *CURRENT CHANGE* THAT PRODUCED THE MAGNETIC VARIATION.

It should be clear now, that an inductor attempts to oppose a change in current flow by producing a back EMF. This property is defined as **inductance**. The symbol for inductance is L. The unit of inductance is the **henry,** and a coil is said to have one henry of inductance when a current change of one ampere causes a back EMF of one volt. The amount of inductance in a coil is influenced by the following factors:

1. Number of turns;
2. Spacing and method of winding;
3. Diameter of the coil;
4. Ratio of diameter to coil length;
5. Type of core.

The type of core refers to the material contained within the center or core of the coil. This may be air, or some easily magnetized substance. A magnetic core has the capability of concentrating and therefore increasing the density of the flux lines of force within the coil, thus increasing the inductance of the coil. Iron sheets or filings are often used for this purpose.

PHASE RELATIONSHIP IN AN INDUCTOR

When a resistance is connected to a source of AC voltage, the current through the resistor is in phase with the applied voltage (Figure 5-4). When voltage is zero, current flow is zero. When voltage is maximum, current is maximum. The same is *not* true when an inductor is substituted for the resistor.

Let us suppose an AC voltage is placed across a coil. At the instant current starts to flow, the following three things occur almost simultaneously:

1. Current starts to increase.

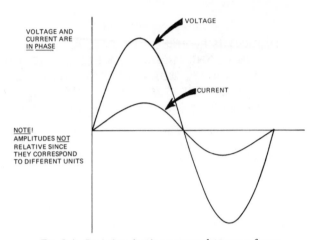

Fig. 5-4: Resistive circuit current-voltage waveforms

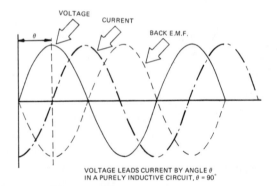

Fig. 5-5: Current and voltage waveforms in an inductive circuit

2. A magnetic field radiates outward.

3. Back EMF is produced opposing the current-flow change in (1).

As a result, the applied voltage reaches maximum *before* the current through the coil. In a purely inductive circuit, the phase difference produced between voltage and current is 90°; voltage leads current by 90°. Figure 5-5 shows the graphical relationship; compare it to Figure 5-4.

INDUCTIVE REACTANCE

Although the property of opposing a change in current flow is termed **inductance**, the actual opposition afforded by a coil is called **inductive reactance**. It is measured in ohms and is given the symbol X_L. Inductive reactance can be calculated using the formula:

$$X_L = 2\pi \, FL$$

where X_L = inductive reactance (ohm);
2π = a constant (π = 3.14);
F = the frequency of the applied voltage; and
L = inductance of the coil (henries)

Note that, once a coil is constructed, the only variable capable of changing X_L is the frequency of the applied signal.

SELF AND MUTUAL INDUCTANCE

We have seen that a coil can have a current (or voltage) induced into it by the moving magnetic field produced by changes of current in the coil itself. Such action of a coil produces a back EMF and is referred to as **self-induction.**

When two coils are placed close together, one with an alternating current passing through it and the other with no prime power source, a current flow is induced into the second coil and its associated circuit. This action occurs because of the cutting of the secondary coil by the constantly expanding and collapsing magnetic field of the first or primary coil, cutting the secondary coil and inducing a current flow into it. This phenomenon is called **mutual inductance** or **transformer action** (Figure 5-6).

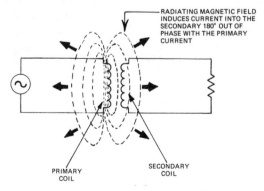

RADIATING MAGNETIC FIELD INDUCES CURRENT INTO THE SECONDARY 180° OUT OF PHASE WITH THE PRIMARY CURRENT

PRIMARY COIL

SECONDARY COIL

Fig. 5-6: Transformer action – by mutual induction

PRACTICAL POINTS ABOUT INDUCTORS

Power Losses

Since inductors consist of wire coils and wire has some resistance, when current flows through an inductor some energy is lost. This is termed **copper loss**. Iron ore coils have two losses in addition to copper losses:

1. **Hysteresis loss:** energy lost in reversing the magnetic field of the core as the current flows through the coil alternates.
2. **Eddy-current loss:** current induced in the iron core by the field around the coil. These currents flow back and forth in the iron and dissipate energy in the form of heat.

Typical Inductors

Inductors fall into three main groups according to the frequency at which they are designated to function:

1. Power frequencies;
2. Audio frequencies;
3. Radio frequencies.

Testing Inductors

An inductor can be tested with an ohmmeter by placing it across the two terminals of the coil and measuring resistance. Coil resistances are given by the manufacturer. If the measured value compares favorably with this given value, the inductor is probably good. If infinite resistance is measured, the coil is open. Any reading 20 percent or more below the manufacturer's value indicates that a number of turns are shorted together. In the case of an iron core coil, always check the resistance from each terminal to the core itself, to determine whether or not a winding has been shorted to the core.

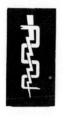

AC circuits II

CHAPTER 6

CAPACITORS AND CAPACITANCE

We learned in the previous chapter that reactors are divided into two classes: (1) those storing energy in an electromagnetic field (**inductors**); and (2) those storing energy in an electrostatic field (**capacitors**). Although both store energy, the methods by which they accomplish this task are entirely different.

A **capacitor** consists of two thin sheets of conducting material or layer of insulating material separated by a small space. Each of the plates, as they are called, is attached by a wire conductor to the circuit of which the capacitor is a part. If a DC voltage source is for an instant connected to the two leads—positive to one, negative to the other—the instant the final connection is made a current will flow for a brief moment only (Figure 6-1). The

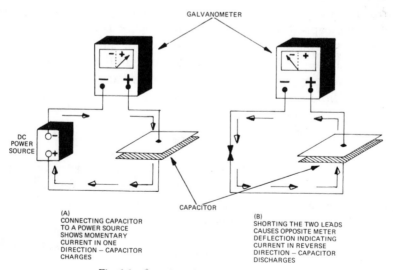

GALVANOMETER

DC POWER SOURCE

CAPACITOR

(A)
CONNECTING CAPACITOR
TO A POWER SOURCE
SHOWS MOMENTARY
CURRENT IN ONE
DIRECTION — CAPACITOR
CHARGES

(B)
SHORTING THE TWO LEADS
CAUSES OPPOSITE METER
DEFLECTION INDICATING
CURRENT IN REVERSE
DIRECTION — CAPACITOR
DISCHARGES

Fig. 6-1: Capacitor charging and discharging

momentary current flow can be detected by connecting a galvanometer into the circuit as shown. Disconnecting the leads from the battery and shorting the two ends together (as in Figure 6-1*B*), will produce another momentary current flow, but this time in the *opposite* direction. From the above experiments, it becomes apparent that the two plates have retained energy while disconnected from the voltage source and later returned it to the circuit.

Let us examine how this was accomplished.

The instant the wires are connected to the DC voltage source the circuit is completed and a path for current exists. The wire connected to the positive terminal of the source feels a deficiency of electrons; therefore, electrons begin to pass from the wire to the positive terminal. This creates a deficiency in the wire that is reflected along its length to the plate and the plate then becomes deficient in electrons; that is, it is charged positively. The opposite phenomenon occurs at the other plate, which becomes negatively charged (excess of electrons). With this charge pattern on the plates, the molecules in the air or other material between the plates feel a distorting force. The electron orbits of these molecules become distorted by the pulling of electrons toward the positive plate and repulsion of them from the negative plate. This distortion of the substance (in this case, air) between the plates helps the capacitor hold its charge (Figure 6-2). The material between the plates is called the **dielectric**; and the amount of charge that can be held by a capacitor at a given voltage is directly related to the type of dielectric used, as well as other factors. The ability to hold charge is termed **capacitance** and is determined by:

1. Area of the plates;
2. Distance between the plates;
3. Type of dielectric used.

The electron orbits of some materials can be distorted much more easily than the orbits of other materials. This fact gives rise to a property assigned to each dielectric material called its **dielectric constant**. Air is used as a reference and is given the value of 1. Mica has a value of 6. This means that if air and mica capacitors of the same dimensions are connected to the same voltage source, the mica capacitor will store 6 times as much

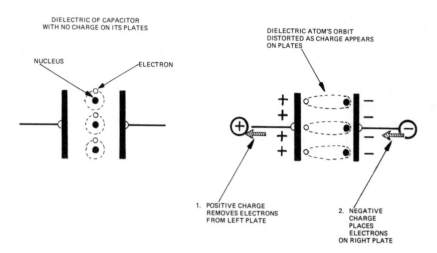

DIELECTRIC OF CAPACITOR
WITH NO CHARGE ON ITS PLATES

NUCLEUS

ELECTRON

DIELECTRIC ATOM'S ORBIT
DISTORTED AS CHARGE APPEARS
ON PLATES

1. POSITIVE CHARGE
REMOVES ELECTRONS
FROM LEFT PLATE

2. NEGATIVE
CHARGE
PLACES
ELECTRONS
ON RIGHT PLATE

Fig. 6-2: How a capacitor holds a charge (adapted from Air Force manual 101-8, radar circuit analysis – modified by the author – courtesy of the United States Air Force)

charge as the air dielectric capacitor. (More current would flow in charging and discharging the mica capacitor.) In short, *the greater the dielectric constant, the greater the capacitance.* The unit of capacitance is the **farad** and it is designated as *the amount of capacitance capable of storing a charge of one coulomb at a potential of one volt.* In practical circuits, the values of capacitance are usually very much smaller than a farad and therefore are expressed in microfarads (1×10^{-6}) (μf) or micromicrofarads (1×10^{-12}) ($\mu\mu$f).

PHASE RELATIONSHIP

At the first instant voltage is applied across a capacitor, maximum current flows in the associated circuit, called the **capacitator charge current.** This current gradually decreases as the capacitor charges, until finally it ceases completely when the capacitor is fully charged. Let us examine why this occurs. At the first instant, the difference between the applied voltage and the potential difference on the capacitor plates is maximum. (The applied voltage is at some positive or negative potential while the plates are at zero potential). Since the difference between the two is maximum, maximum charging current will flow. As the capacitor's plates begin to charge, the voltage between them opposes the applied voltage and the capacitor's voltage. This reduces current flow. This sequence progresses until the capacitor is fully charged ($E_C = E_A$) at which time the back EMF is equal to the applied voltage; hence, the net voltage is zero and no current flows. The overall process is shown by the current and voltage curves in Figure 6-3.

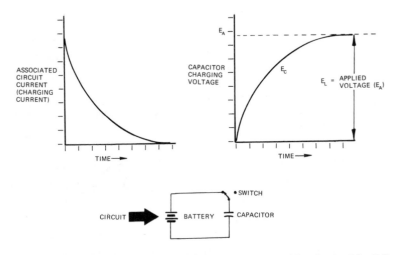

Fig. 6-3:   *Relationship between voltage and current in a capacitive circuit with a DC voltage applied.*

In short, from this example it could be said that in a capacitive circuit, the *current is maximum when the voltage is minimum.*

If the applied voltage is an alternating one, at the time the charge reaches maximum, the applied voltage is also at maximum; it then begins to decrease.

Since the capacitor is charged to a maximum, and the voltage that produced that charge is decreasing, the capacitor must now release some of its charge; in short, it must discharge. The direction of discharge is opposite to the charge path. In other words, the direction of circuit current reverses (Figures 6-4 and 6-5).

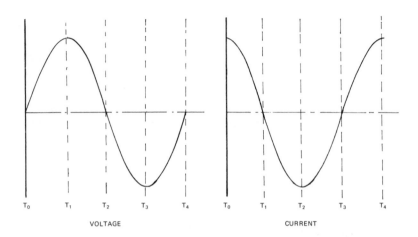

Fig. 6-4: *Graph of capacitor voltage and current in an AC circuit*

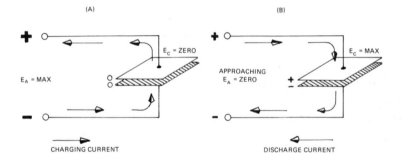

Fig. 6-5: *Diagram showing how capacitive current changes polarity before the applied voltage (i.e., current leads voltage) in an AC circuit*

From Figure 6-6B it can be seen that current always leads voltage in a *capacitive* circuit by 90 degrees. In the discussion of inductors in *inductive* circuits, it was the voltage that led the current. It is a simple matter to remember these two relationships with the help of a memory aid; *ELI, the ICE MAN.* **ELI** refers to *voltage (E)* in an *inductive* circuit *(L)* leading *current (I);* **ICE** refers to *current (I)* in a *capacitive* circuit *(C)* leading *voltage (E).*

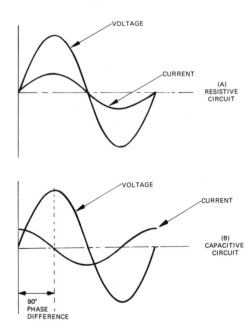

Fig. 6-6: Comparison of resistive and capacitive circuit waveforms

Since current leads voltage in a capacitive circuit, it follows that *a capacitor tends to oppose a change in voltage.* This together with an inductor's property of opposing a change in current flow becomes increasingly useful when the two are combined and used in power supplies to regulate outputs of direct current. This application will be discussed in greater detail in Chapter 19.

CAPACITIVE REACTANCE

The opposition afforded by a capacitor to current flow in an AC circuit is called **capacitive reactance.** It is a result of distorting the molecular structure of the capacitor's dielectric material. The symbol for the property is X_C and it is measured in ohms. The value of X_C is dependent upon the following factors:

1. Capacitance of the capacitor;
2. Frequency of the applied signal;
3. $1/2\pi$, a constant.

The formula for X_C is given as:

$$X_C = 1/2\pi\,FC$$

where X_C = capacitive reactance in ohms
F = frequency in cps
C = capacitance in farads

PRACTICAL POINTS ABOUT CAPACITORS

Power Losses

Since it is impossible to construct a perfect or ideal capacitor, some power is lost or dissipated in every practical capacitor. Capacitor losses are classified as follows:

1. *Resistance loss:* losses due to the resistance of the wires connected to the plates and the plates themselves.
2. *Leakage loss:* losses due to small amounts of current flowing through the dielectric from plate to plate.
3. *Dielectric absorption loss:* energy that is absorbed by the dielectric and *not* given up by the capacitor as it discharges.
4. *Dielectric hysteresis loss:* energy required to reverse the polarity of the electric field existing across the plates of a capacitor.

Voltage Ratings

These voltage figures indicate the maximum continual and surge values a capacitor can handle.

1. *DC working voltage:* maximum DC voltage that a capacitor can withstand under continuous operation at normal operating temperature.
2. *Peak voltage:* maximum peak value of AC voltage the capacitor can withstand continually under normal operating temperature.
3. *Surge voltage:* maximum voltage that can be tolerated for five minutes.

Testing Capacitors

A paper capacitor can be tested with an ohmmeter by measuring the resistance between its two terminals. An infinite reading means the capacitor is probably good. Anything less than infinity means the dielectric is damaged and the capacitor is probably useless.

When electrolytic (polarized) capacitors are tested this way, they will indicate a short momentarily. Then the needle should slowly rise to about 1 megohm. Anything less than 1 megohm indicates probable damage to the oxide coating.

In addition to the common electrolytic capacitors (for use with DC only) there are many other types of capacitors available in a wide variety of shapes, sizes, and dielectric materials. The most commonly encountered are (1) dry electrolytic paper capacitors, (2) wet electrolytic film capacitors; (3) mica capacitors, and (4) ceramic capacitors. The latter two types are most often manufactured as (relatively) small, square, rectangular, or flat, round, molded units, while the first two types are metal or paper-encased cylinders or square metal-covered devices.

AC circuits III

CHAPTER 7

REACTANCE AND IMPEDANCE

When the properties of *inductive reactance, capacitive react-ance,* and *resistance* are all present in one circuit, the overall opposition to any alternating current in that circuit becomes a complex function of the three properties combined, and not just a simple sum of their individual effects.

This is not difficult to understand when one remembers that the opposition of a reactor to current flow varies as the voltage or current varies. For example, an *inductor* shows no opposition to a direct current except that pure resistance of the wire from which it is made. However, if an alternating current is passed through the wire, as the frequency of the AC increases, the inductive reactance increases. The total opposition to current of such an RL circuit then becomes a function of *R, L,* and the frequency.

The total opposition to current flow in a *resistive-reactive* circuit (RL, RC or RLC) is called **impedance** (symbol, *Z*). Impedance is measured in *ohms* and is calculated by using the circuit values of R, X_L, and/or X_C. The formula for impedance (Z) in an *RL* (resistive-inductive) circuit is:

$$Z = \sqrt{R^2 + X_L^2}$$

where R = resistance (ohms)
X_L = inductive reactance (ohms)

In a circuit with resistance and capacitance (an RC circuit), the formula for impedance is similar:

$$Z = \sqrt{R^2 + X_C^2}$$

When all three properties are combined in a circuit, the evaluation of Z becomes a little more difficult and the following two formulas are used:

$$Z = \sqrt{R^2 + (X_L - X_C)^2} \qquad \text{When } X_L > X_C$$

or, $$Z = \sqrt{R^2 + (X_C - X_L)^2} \qquad \text{When } X_C > X_L$$

Inductive reactance can be subtracted from capacitive reactance and vice versa, since their effects when plotted as vectors are 180° out of phase with each other. (Remember *ELI–ICE*). In an inductive circuit, voltage *leads* current; in a capacitive circuit, voltage *lags* current. Since it is the opposition to current flow that produces these voltages, the reactances can be assigned the same phase angles as their respective voltages (Figure 7-1). Resistance is referenced at zero degrees because there is no phase difference between the current through a resistor and the voltage across it. (As voltage increases, so does current and vice versa.)

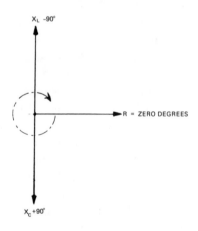

Fig. 7-1: Reactances in a resistive-capacitive-inductive circuit

An AC circuit can be analyzed once circuit impedance has been determined, by using Ohm's Law, in the form: $E_T = I_T \times R_T$ and replacing R with Z to give $E_T = I_T \times Z$.

RESONANCE

We have seen that both X_L and X_C are frequency-dependent. It has also been shown that as frequency increases, X_L increases but X_C decreases; and as frequency decreases, X_L decreases and X_C increases. In brief, X_L is directly proportional to the applied frequency, while X_C is inversely proportional to the applied frequency. From this information we can conclude that in a circuit containing both L and C, there will be some frequency, at which $X_C = X_L$. The formula for finding this frequency, designated **resonant frequency** (F_r), can be obtained as follows:

1. Since $X_C = X_L$

2. But $X_L = 2\pi\,\text{FL}$ and $X_C = \dfrac{1}{2\pi\,\text{FC}}$

3. Then $2\pi\,\text{FL} = \dfrac{1}{2\pi\,\text{FC}}$

4. And $(F_r)^2 = \dfrac{1}{4\pi^2\,\text{LC}}$

5. Or, taking the square root, $F_r = \dfrac{1}{2\pi\sqrt{\text{LC}}}$

It should be noted that *above F_r* a circuit containing both L and C will act *inductively* while *below F_r* it will act *capacitively*. At F_r, however, the circuit functions as a pure resistance since the effects of X_L and X_C are equal and 180° out of phase and thus cancel each other.

RESONANT FILTERS

An example of the application of the concept of circuit resonance is found in filter circuits.

Resonant filter circuits are used to obtain either selective rejection or selective acceptance of signals falling within a prescribed narrow band of frequencies. As we have seen, every reactive circuit has its own resonant frequency, and at that frequency, X_L and X_C are equal and opposite, resulting in a cancellation of their effects. This cancellation leaves only the circuit resistance to oppose current. If we place such a reactive circuit either (a) in series, or (b) in parallel with the load to be driven, current to the load can be selectively controlled. These applications are described in the following paragraphs and shown in Figure 7-2.

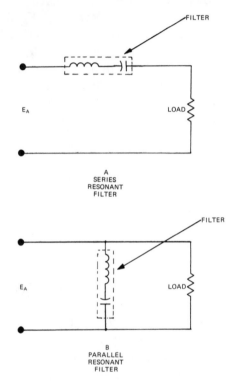

Fig. 7-2: Filter circuits used to control load current.

1. *Series resonant filters (band pass)* are placed in series with the load so that at reasonance *maximum* current is passed to the load.
2. *Parallel resonant filters (band reject)* are placed in parallel with the load so that at resonance *minimum* current flows through the load and maximum current through the resonant circuit.

Resonant filter circuits are used in many medical instrument applications in which the physiological signal being detected falls within a narrow band of frequencies. One important example is in electrocardiographic (ECG) instruments, in which special filter circuits are used to remove 60 hertz (Hz) interference.

R.C. TIME CONSTANTS

The time it takes for a capacitor to charge to an applied voltage is determined by two factors: (1) the size of the capacitor, and (2) the size of the circuit resistance through which the charging current must pass. During the charging process, the greater the accumulated charge on the capacitor, the weaker the charging current. Since the charging current passes through the resistor, the voltage across the resistor varies in proportion to that current ($E = I \times R$). Figure 7-3 shows the related wave forms in an RC series circuit to which a square wave input has been applied.

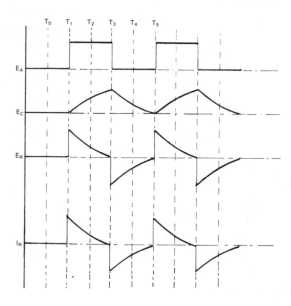

Fig. 7-3: RC circuit voltage – current waveforms

At T_1 the applied voltage instantaneously goes to maximum and E_c, the accumulated charge in the capacitor, is zero. The capacitor starts to charge; therefore, maximum charge current flows. That current passes through R, and consequently the voltage across R at

T_1 is maximum. At T_2 the capacitor has become partially charged and this results in a decrease in charge current which in turn causes less voltage drop across R. (Notice that at all times $E_C + E_R = E_A$, satisfying the rule for voltage in a series circuit.) At T_3 the capacitor reaches its maximum charge state and E_A is reduced to zero. As a result the charging current is zero and the voltage across R is also zero. Immediately the capacitor starts to discharge. Maximum discharge current now flows in the *opposite* direction (relative to the direction of the charge current). Once again a maximum voltage will be felt across R, but opposite in polarity to the capacitor voltage ($E_C + E_R = E_A$ still holds true: maximum positive + maximum negative = 0). The steadily decreasing discharge current continues until at T_5 the charge across the capacitor is zero, E_R is zero, and current is zero. By examining the waveforms for E_A and E_C, it becomes easier to see how a capacitor tends to oppose change in voltage. E_A goes to a maximum rapidly, while E_C progresses slowly upward. When E_A drops to zero rapidly, E_C drops slowly to zero.

In order for a capacitor to charge to the approximate full value of the applied voltage, or to discharge completely, a certain period of time is needed. This period is equal to five times a quantity known as the **time constant** of the capacitor. The time constant is the time required for a capacitor to charge to 63.2 per cent of E_A or to discharge to 36.8 per cent of the original E_C. A capacitor never actually charges to one hundred per cent of E_A, but for practical purposes it is considered to be fully charged after five time constants. Figure 7-4 shows a universal, time constant charge/discharge chart.

The actual time it takes a capacitor to reach its fully charged condition is determined by the size of the capacitor, and the circuit resistance through which the charging current passes. The formula $T = RC$ gives the time constant in seconds.

> **Example:** If we have a circuit capacitance of 10 microfarads and a resistance of 5 megohms, the capacitor will charge to 63.2 per cent of an applied voltage in $(5 \times 10^6)(10 \times 10^{-6}) = 50$ seconds. By decreasing the size of R to 5 kilohms, the time constant is shortened to $(5 \times 10^3)(10 \times 10^{-6}) = 50 \times 10^{-3}$ seconds or 50 milli-

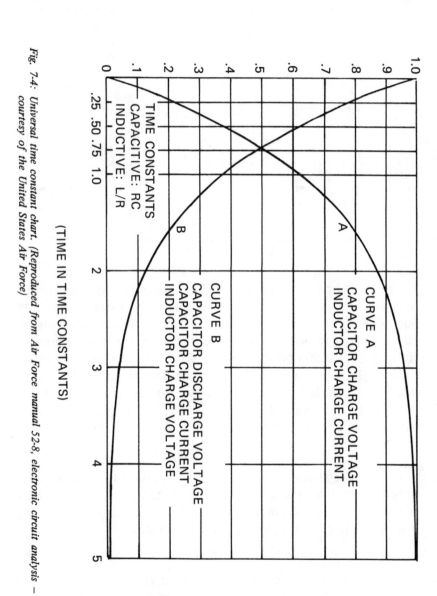

Fig. 7-4: Universal time constant chart. (Reproduced from Air Force manual 52-8, electronic circuit analysis – courtesy of the United States Air Force)

seconds. Graphing the two capacitor charge curves would give results approximating those shown in Figure 7-5.

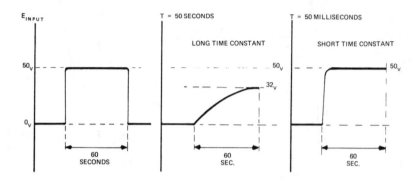

Fig. 7-5: Circuit time constant and its effect on an input signal

From this brief examination, it should be apparent to the reader that *RC* circuits can be designed to selectively distort waveforms. Such circuits are termed **waveshaping circuits.** The circuit with T = 50 seconds is referred to as a *long time constant circuit* and the circuit with T = 50 milliseconds as a *short time constant circuit.*

In addition to waveshaping, *RC* circuits can be used as filters (mentioned earlier in this chapter) or as coupling circuits (effectively blocking DC potentials, but allowing AC signals to pass). These circuits will be discussed in more detail later.

RL TIME CONSTANTS

Just as a capacitor requires one time constant to reach a charge condition of 63.2 per cent of E_A, an inductor requires one time constant to reach the point at which 63.2 per cent I_{MAX} is flowing through it. The formula for an *RL* time constant is

$$T = L/R$$

Figure 7-6 shows the waveforms in an *RL* circuit to which a square wave voltage has been applied. Assuming the applied signal to be the same as that applied to the RC circuit in the previous section, let us examine the result.

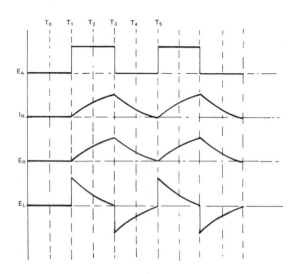

Fig. 7-6: RL circuit voltage — current waveforms

At T_1, E_A goes rapidly to maximum. Circuit current cannot rise immediately to maximum because it is retarded by the back EMF of the inductor. Since the voltage across the resistor is determined by the current through it, and at T_1, I is zero, then E_R at T_1 is also zero. However, because $E_R + E_L = E_A$ must also be true, at T_1 maximum voltage is felt across the inductor (E_L). At T_2 current flow has increased, E_R has proportionately increased, and E_L has decreased. At T_3, E_A goes to zero. Current through the inductor attempts to go to zero, but is instead maintained by the collapsing magnetic field. E_R follows the current, slowly decreasing as I decreases. The negative segment of the inductor waveform at T_3 is due to the initial back EMF of the coil when E_A suddenly goes to zero. As current through the coil decreases to zero, the inductor voltage also decreases to zero. Notice that at T_3 with $E_A = 0$, E_R = positive and E_L = negative; therefore, $E_R + E_L = E_A$. Once more the rule for voltage in a series circuit is maintained.

DIFFERENTIATION AND INTEGRATION

The mathematical operations of differentiating and integrating can be accomplished employing RC and RL circuits. Although the result is not exact due to the limitations of practical circuit construction and response, a very close approximate result can generally be obtained. Such circuits find diverse application in computers and in many types of biomedical instrumentation.

When one differentiates mathematically, it is analogous to finding the instantaneous rate at which something changes. For example, finding the rate at which the curve shown in Figure 7-7 is changing at each instant would be finding a derivative. We would be differentiating the function represented by the curve.

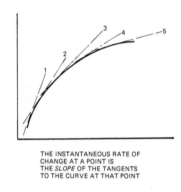

THE INSTANTANEOUS RATE OF
CHANGE AT A POINT IS
THE *SLOPE* OF THE TANGENTS
TO THE CURVE AT THAT POINT

Fig. 7-7: Differentiating a curve mathematically

One of the simplest and most common differentiating circuits used in instrumentation is an *RC* circuit. Figure 7-8 shows a typical differentiator circuit, with the output taken across the resistor.

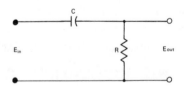

Fig. 7-8: An RC differentiating circuit

Referring to Figure 7-9, the input (A) to such an RC differentiator is a square wave. At T_1, E_A goes almost instantaneously to maximum. The derivative of this signal (B) is very large at that instant because the voltage is rising very rapidly. When the voltage reaches its maximum and then remains constant until T_2, the derivative is zero because the voltage is *not changing*. At T_2 the voltage goes sharply *down;* therefore, the derivative goes to a large *negative* value. As the voltage remains *unchanged* for an interval, the derivative again becomes zero, and so on.

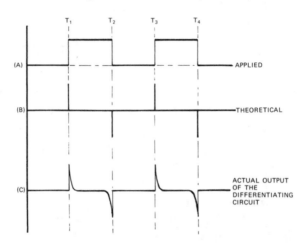

Fig. 7-9: Theoretical versus actual differentiation

Curve *(B)* shows these sharp positive and negative peaks and the zero values between them. The actual output of the differentiating circuit would look something like curve *(C)*, which is a fairly close approximation of *(B)*.

The time constant for a differentiator must be short, enabling the capacitor to charge rapidly. It should be less than or equal to 0.2 of the time required for one cycle of the input.

The circuit pictured in Figure 7-8 can also be modified to function as an integrator by reversing the position of the components, changing their relative values, and taking the output not from the resistor but from across the capacitor. An integrating circuit performs the opposite function to that of a differentiator. The circuit *averages* the value of an input signal over a period of time. Finding the area under the curve shown in Figure 7-10 is an example of the mathematical process of integration.

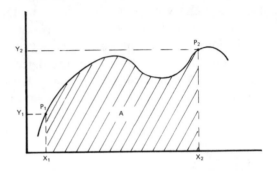

Fig. 7-10: Finding the area under a curve—an example of integration

An example of electronic integration utilizing an RC circuit can be seen by referring to Figure 7-11. The input signal (E_A) is positive going from T_1 to T_2. From T_2 to T_3 it is negative. The integrated waveshape at T_1 therefore begins to go positive (or add) at a constant rate, while at T_2 it begins to go negative (or subtract) at a constant rate. The result is that waveform E_C represents the *average* value of E_A from T_1 to T_3.

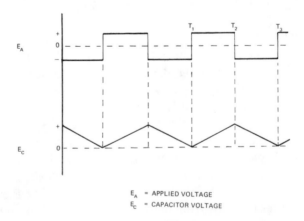

E_A = APPLIED VOLTAGE
E_C = CAPACITOR VOLTAGE

Fig. 7-11: Electronic integration of a square wave

The time constant for an integrating circuit must be a long one, enabling the capacitor to charge and discharge early on its charge curve and therefore at a linear rate. Its value must be at least 20 times the period of the input.

The two circuits just described are very simple forms of integrating and differentiating networks; much more complex circuits exist. However, all integrating circuits find much use in instrumentation converting various forms of analog signals (such as curves from recorders) into digital values that may be read directly off an instrument's display module.

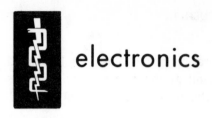 electronics

CHAPTER 8

ELECTRON EMISSION

From a simple pH meter, to a complex heart rate computer, a unit of electronic equipment, whatever its function, consists of *five* basic components in various circuit combinations, numbers, and arrangements. These fundamental components are **resistors, inductors, capacitors, vacuum tubes,** and **semiconductors.** To date we have studied the first three; we will now begin the study of vacuum tubes, followed by an examination of semiconductors.

In 1883, Thomas Edison discovered the first vacuum tube phenomenon. While he was experimenting with an evacuated glass bulb containing a wire filament and a metal plate, he noticed that when the wire filament was heated and a positive potential was applied to the metal plate, a current flowed in the external circuit. In brief, he had discovered that certain metals when heated emit electrons, and that these electrons are attracted through space by a charged body.

This phenomenon, **electron emission,** is the fundamental concept upon which the operation of the vacuum tube is based.

Types of Emission

The electron emission discovered by Edison can be likened to the effects produced when water is boiled. As water temperature is increased by the application of heat, some water molecules are able to overcome intermolecular bonds, break free, and become steam or vapor molecules. In the same way, as heat is applied to some materials, the vibrational or kinetic energy of some electrons is increased to the point that electrons tear themselves free from the mother system to be attracted to a positive charge. The type of emission that requires the introduction of heat is termed **thermionic emission.**

78

Another form of electron emission employs the use of a high difference of potential to release electrons. We know from an earlier discussion that some electrons within metals are "free" in that they are not bound to any particular atom. These electrons are easily attracted by large electrostatic charges. A strong electrostatic field can be used to pull these electrons off an emitting material, if the attractive force (electric field) is greater than the binding force. This type of emission is also known as **electrostatic** or **cold-cathode emission**, and is more easily accomplished if the emitter has a pointed contour or a rough surface.

A **photon** is a discrete unit of light energy and it too can be made to produce electron emission. A special class of substances known as photosensitive materials will emit electrons when struck by light energy, and the process is known as **photoemission**. Some materials falling in this class are cesium, germanium, and sodium. Vacuum tubes containing photosensitive elements are used as light-detecting devices in a large number of analytical instruments, such as colorimeters, spectrophotometers, etc. In addition, many other instruments employ **photoelectric cells**, which are semiconductors made from photosensitive materials.

The final type of electron emission to be considered is called **secondary emission**. This form of emission is brought about by the action of high velocity particles (e.g., electrons) moving through space and then striking another substance, causing other electrons to be "knocked off." One can compare this action to a bullet hitting a wall and causing a shower of stone fragments to be "emitted."

In summary, it may be said that any means by which an electron is caused to leave a material and pass into space is classed as emission, and in order to produce emission, some form of energy input is required.

THE DIODE

Diode is a combination of two word fragments: *di*, meaning two, and *ode* from electrode. Simply put, a diode is a two-electrode (or element) vacuum tube. The "emitter," or source of electrons, is called the **cathode**, and the "collector" is called the **plate**. Three types of materials serve the purpose of emitters: (1)

tungsten, (2) thoriated tungsten, and (3) earth oxides. Their properties are summarized in Table 8-1.

TABLE 8-1

PROPERTIES OF CATHODE EMITTING MATERIALS

Material	Physical Strength	Operating Temperature	Efficiency	General Use
Tungsten	Rugged	High	Low	High Power Tubes
Thoriated tungsten	Medium	Medium	Medium	Medium Power Tubes
Earth oxides	Fragile	Low	High	Low Power Tubes

Most vacuum tubes employ thermionic emission brought about by either (1) direct or (2) indirect heating of the cathode. When comparing directly and indirectly heated cathodes, it has been found that an AC signal applied to a directly heated cathode yields a variation in the current used to heat the element which in turn varies the number of electrons emitted (they come off in "waves"). Such variation in emission produces "tube noise." With the use of an indirectly heated cathode, the heater element or filament is in close proximity to the cathode. After reaching operating temperature, the filament gives off heat at a relatively stable rate, and keeps the cathode at a steady temperature which in turn produces a relatively uniform rate of boil-off of electrons.

The physical construction of the diode is shown in Figure 8-1 and schematic diagrams are shown in Figure 8-2.

The filament or heater is inserted in a glass base, and the cathode is placed around it. The plate (or anode) is then placed around them both. The whole assembly is finally inserted into a glass envelope which is evacuated (air removed) and then sealed.

Theory of Operation

The operation of a vacuum tube utilizes the fact that like charges repel and unlike charges attract. Since electrons are

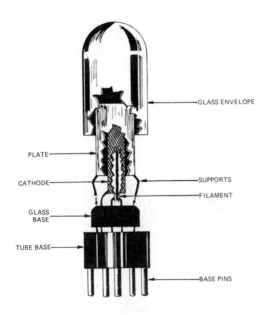

Fig. 8-1: Exploded view of a diode vacuum tube

charged negatively, as soon as they are emitted from the cathode they will be attracted by a positively charged plate and a current will flow in the external circuit. A negatively charged plate will repel these electrons, resulting in no circuit current. When filament power is applied, electrons form a cloud or "space-charge" in the vicinity of the cathode. By varying the potential on the plate, we

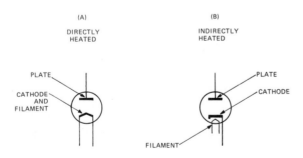

Fig. 8-2: Vacuum tube diode schematic symbols

can cause more or fewer of these electrons to carry current through the tube.

Figure 8-3 illustrates this action. Notice that when the cathode is at a relatively positive potential (with respect to the plate) the electrons are attracted back to the cathode and no current flows. Thus the basic principle of vacuum tube operation is *unidirectional current flow.*

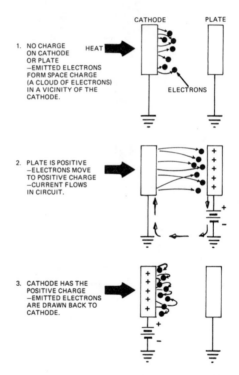

Fig. 8-3: Current flow through a tube. (Courtesy Philco-Ford Corp., Tech. Rep. Division, Fort Washington, Penna.) — modified by the author

The Characteristic Curve

The current flowing in the anode circuit of a vacuum tube diode is designated **plate current**. It is apparent that as the potential on the plate of a diode is increased, more of the emitted electrons will flow to the plate. By plotting a graph of plate voltage (E_p) versus plate current (I_p), a curve is developed which is characteristic for the particular type of diode tested. As shown in Figure 8-4, the curve will show an increase of plate current for an increase in plate voltage. This continues until a leveling off point is reached and a further increase in E_p produces no change (increase) in I_p. At this point, designated as **saturation**, all electrons emitted by the cathode are being drawn to the plate. However, if the tube's heater temperature is increased, then more electrons become available due to increased emission and I_p will increase. Figure 8-4 shows an E_p I_p characteristic curve for two heater temperatures.

> NOTE: The characteristic curve shows how much of a charge in plate current occurs for a given change in plate voltage.

When there is a difference of potential between the cathode and the plate of a diode causing current to flow, it can be regarded as a "voltage drop" across the tube. Since there *is* a voltage drop, there must also be (according to Ohm's Law) some value of resistance across which the EMF is dropped. This "tube resistance" is known as the **plate resistance** of the tube. Its value can be calculated by taking the E_p I_p values at any point on the E_p I_p curve and substituting in Ohm's Law: $R = E/I$.

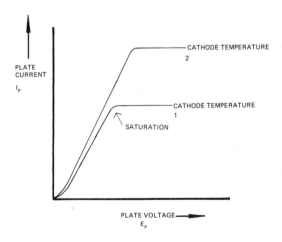

Fig. 8-4: E_pI_p characteristic curves for two cathode temperatures.

Application of Diodes

Since a diode is a unidirectional current device, it is admirably suited to changing an AC voltage to a DC voltage. This action is called **rectification**, and Figure 8-5 illustrates the operation of a typical diode rectifier.

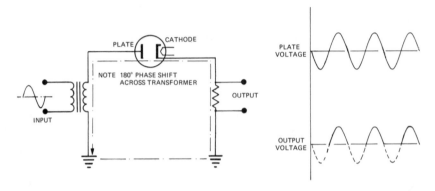

Fig. 8-5: A diode functioning as a half-wave rectifier (broken line indicates current path)

On the first (negative) half cycle of the signal at the transformer's secondary winding, the plate of the tube is negative with respect to the cathode; consequently no current can flow through the tube circuit and the output generated will be zero. However, on the second, or positive, half cycle of the signal, the plate is positive with respect to the cathode. This results in current flow through the tube, and therefore an output occurs. On the subsequent negative half cycle, the initial action is repeated and once more no output voltage is generated. Note that the original input is reversed in phase by the transformer. This overall process is known as **half wave rectification** as only half of the input is reproduced in the output. By placing diodes into a circuit as shown in Figure 8-6, **full wave rectification** is obtained. On one half cycle V_1, its plate being positive, conducts, while V_2 with a negative plate does not, and current flows up through R_L producing an output. On the other half cycle V_1 does not conduct since its plate is now negative, but V_2 conducts and current again flows up through R_L yielding the second half of the output.

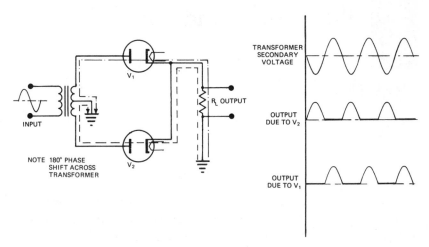

Fig. 8-6: A full-wave rectifier using two diodes (broken lines indicate current paths)

Although the primary use of diodes is rectification, they are used in many other applications; all, however, are based on the principle of unidirectional current flow.

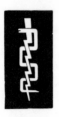 the triode and amplification

CHAPTER 9

THE TRIODE

The second type of vacuum tube to be developed was the **triode**. Once again, the name is a compound word meaning a vacuum tube with three elements. The first two electrodes are familiar: the *cathode* and the *plate*. The third is a wire assembly known commonly as the *control grid*. The grid is placed between the plate and the cathode to control electron flow through the tube. It is placed physically closer to the cathode than the plate and the reason for this will become apparent as we study the theory of operation of a triode.

Physical Construction and Schematic Symbols

Figure 9-1 shows a sectional view of a triode. Notice that the grid, although located *between* the plate and cathode, is con-

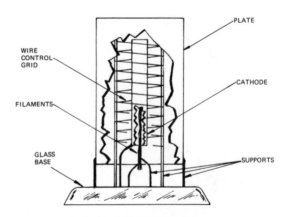

Fig. 9-1: Cut-away view of the elements of a triode tube

86

structed so that electrons can pass freely from the cathode to the plate.

Grids can be wound in a number of different ways, but all types function in the same way. The grid may be made of any of the following materials: molybdenum, nichrome, iron, nickel, tungsten, or tantalum.

It is important to note that grids operate at low enough temperatures so as **not** to function as emitters.

A triode tube is usually represented by a schematic diagram as shown in Figure 9-2.

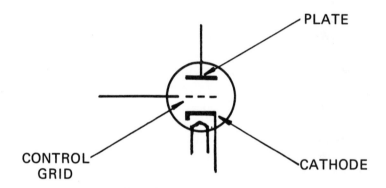

Fig. 9-2: Schematic representation of a triode tube

Theory of Triode Operation

The grid is used for the express purpose of controlling the electron flow through the tube and is thus referred to as the **control grid**. During normal operation the grid potential *with reference to the cathode* is usually varied continually. This varying potential has a changing effect upon electrons emitted by the cathode (and attracted to the plate) as they come into the vicinity of the grid. The final outcome is control of the tube's plate current by the grid voltage. Let us examine three ways in which the grid potential (always taken with respect to the cathode) can affect plate current. In the following examples, the cathode is connected directly to ground, so the grid potential is taken with respect to ground.

Zero Control Grid Voltage: Zero control grid voltage can be obtained by either connecting the grid to ground or by leaving the grid loose or "floating" (no connection). In the first instance, as electrons pass from cathode to plate through the grid, some of them strike the grid and become fixed in its molecular structure. An accumulation of electrons builds up on the grid and it becomes slightly negative (with respect to ground). This results in a current flow from the grid to ground, and this *grid current* can affect tube efficiency.

In the second instance, (with no connection on the grid) the electrons striking the grid continue to accumulate, making the grid more and more negative until it reaches a negative potential that is capable of overcoming the plate's positive attraction, thereby completely stopping or "cutting off" plate current.

Thus, these two means of applying zero potential to a grid have acutely different effects on plate current.

Positive Control Grid Voltage: A positive voltage applied to the control grid acts to accelerate electrons traveling to the plate and hence increases their flow. Application of a *fixed* positive grid voltage is used only in special cases, since the point may be reached at which the positive grid begins to attract more electrons that it allows to pass to the plate. Thus, plate current decreases while grid current increases. This may lead to destruction of the tube as too much current may flow through the grid element. (A method of limiting this current will be discussed later).

In a triode vacuum tube's normal operation, there exists a condition in which a positive potential applied to the grid is not of enough magnitude to cause a heavy grid current to flow, but is still of a high enough value to exhibit no further increase in plate current should grid voltage increase further. This condition is known as *saturation,* and is due to the fact that all the electrons emitted by the cathode are being attracted either to the plate or the grid. Consequently an increase in either grid or plate voltage will not increase plate current any further.

Negative Control Grid Voltage: The grid of a triode is usually operated at a voltage slightly negative with respect to the cathode, since even with a negative potential on the grid, electrons are still able to pass to the plate because of the grid's loose structure. A small negative value on the grid tends to repel electrons trying to pass to the plate, thereby limiting the number reaching the plate. If this negative value is gradually increased (made more negative), it eventually reaches some point at which all the electrons are repelled and no plate current flows. This condition is known as *cut-off.*

The amount of negative voltage required *on the grid* to reach cut-off is much smaller in magnitude than the amount of positive voltage *on the plate* that would be required to overcome the cut-off condition. Thus it can be seen that, due to the proximity of the grid to the cathode, the grid has greater control over plate current than does the plate voltage.

Limiting Grid Current

The amount of current that flows through the grid to ground can be limited by placing a very large resistance in the grid lead circuit, usually in the area of 5-6 megohms. This value of resistance limits current flow, but does not affect the grid's control of plate current.

AMPLIFICATION

Amplification is the process of boosting the amplitude or strength of an electrical signal. The signal to be amplified is used to control a much larger system in such a way as to reproduce itself at the output with a value many times the original.

Triodes find their major application as amplifiers although, as will be seen in later chapters, they can be used in many other types of circuits.

No matter what the designation of a particular amplifier may be (*i.e.,* power amplifier, audio amplifier, etc.), the process of amplification is basically the same in all cases, and understanding how a simple amplifier works serves as a basis for understanding all types of amplifiers.

Let us examine the process in more detail (Figure 9-3, *A*).

Assume we have the following situation:

1. An input signal which varies 2 volts positive and 2 volts negative.
2. A triode amplifier having an ambient (or zero grid voltage)

current flow of 20 ma, which will vary by 5 ma, for each change of 2 volts on the grid. (This characteristic response is dictated by the tube design).

3. A 5 KΩ resistor in series with the tube, such that the total voltage available (200 volts) is dropped across the tube and the resistor.

With no input on the grid, the current through the tube and the resistor is 20 ma. In this case the voltage across R is 100 volts. $E = I \times R = (20) \times (5) = 100$. Accordingly, the remaining 100 volts must be dropped across the tube. The voltage then at point A, with respect to ground, is 100 volts.

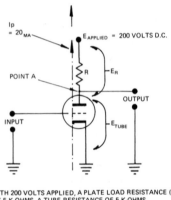

WITH 200 VOLTS APPLIED, A PLATE LOAD RESISTANCE (R)
OF 5 K-OHMS, A TUBE RESISTANCE OF 5 K-OHMS,
AND NO INPUT, THE PLATE CURRENT IS A STEADY
20 MILLIAMPS, THE OUTPUT A STEADY 100 VOLTS.

Fig. 9-3(A): Triode – fixed operating values

When the input signal is applied to the grid of the tube (Figure 9-3, *B*), the following occurs:

1. As the input signal swings positive, it drives the grid 2 volts positive; referring to the previously stated characteristics we see that current through the tube therefore increases from 20 ma to 25 ma.

2. A current of 25 ma through the plate resistor (5KΩ) changes the voltage dropped across it to 125 volts. This in turn leaves only 75 volts across the tube and the voltage at point A is therefore 75 volts.

3. When the negative portion of the input sends the grid voltage to minus 2 volts, the current through the tube follows, decreasing to 15 ma.

4. A current of 15 ma through the plate resistor (5KΩ) causes the voltage drop across it to become 75 volts, and this leaves 125 volts across the tube. The voltage at point *A* is now 125 volts.

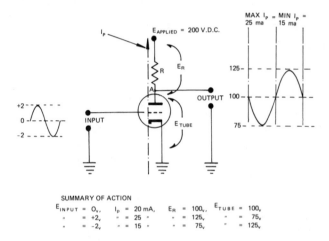

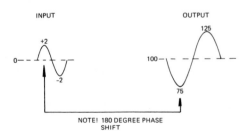

SUMMARY OF ACTION

E_{INPUT} = 0_v, I_p = 20 mA, E_R = 100_v, E_{TUBE} = 100_v
  "   = $+2_v$,   " = 25 "   " = 125_v,   "   = 75_v
  "   = -2_v,   " = 15 "   " = 75_v "   = 125_v

Fig. 9-3(B): Triode – operating as an amplifier

An overview of the whole process (Figure 9-4) shows that the input signal of 4 volts peak to peak (+2/-2v) has produced an output signal varying 50 volts peak to peak (75v/125v). In addition, note that a phase reversal of 180° has occurred between

Fig. 9-4: Comparison of input and output voltages in an amplifier

the input and output signals. The voltage at point A in Figures 9-3(A) and 9-3(B) is called the *plate voltage* (symbol, E_p). The input voltage is called the *grid* voltage (symbol E_g).

The gain or *amplification factor* of an amplifier is obtained by dividing the change in plate voltage by the simultaneous change in grid voltage. In our example, the result is: $E_p/E_g = 50/4 = 12.5$.

AMPLIFIER TYPES BY FUNCTIONAL DESIGNATION

The triode amplifier described in the previous paragraphs of this chapter is the least complex example of many functionally varied amplifiers. Although the fundamental concept of how an amplifier operates is applicable to almost all types of amplifier circuits, differences based on the specific function of an amplifier make for a great variety of types. In the brief summary of various kinds of amplifiers in the following paragraphs, the amplifiers discussed contain more than one tube or stage of amplification. More detailed information concerning them will be found in Section II, Chapters 18 and 19.

The **single-ended amplifier** is the simplest, most common type of amplifier design and is used in a wide variety of electronic devices. The designation *single-ended* comes from the fact that only one input signal is applied to the circuit (between the grid and ground). Single-ended amplifiers are used mostly in relatively simple circuitry in which the operating specifications and requirements of stability, noise rejection, etc., are not too rigid.

The **push-pull amplifier** describes a circuit in which two conventional single-ended amplifiers are hooked in parallel in order to obtain a high gain, or high power, output signal with low distortion. A transformer or phase inverter input circuit is also required with a push-pull amplifier so that the input signal can be split and fed into two grids simultaneously but with opposite phase. The two signals are amplified, and the push-pull output is the sum of the two amplified signals. Because it accepts two inputs, a push-pull amplifier is called a **double-ended amplifier.**

The **differential amplifier** is a special type of double-ended or push-pull amplifier. Differential amplifiers accept two input signals in much the same way as an ordinary push-pull amplifier but, instead of yielding an output signal that is the amplified sum of the two inputs, it gives an output equal to the amplified difference between the two. This operating characteristic makes differential amplifiers useful in noise rejection circuits and also in differential signal detectors.

Chopper amplifiers are used for "chopping" or "modulating" a DC signal into AC or intermittent DC form so that it can be amplified by a conventional amplifier without being distorted by the drift problems common to most DC systems. Consequently, chopper amplifiers are not really amplifiers alone but amplifier systems, made up of (1) a chopper (or modulator), (2) an amplifier, and in some applications (3) a de-chopper (or demodulator).

Operational amplifiers are another type of packaged amplifier system containing more than one stage. They are capable of performing mathematical operations on a signal, or signals (summing, integrating, etc.) as well as almost any conventional amplifier function.

Other kinds of amplifiers often used in medical instrumentation are (1) **buffer amplifiers,** used for impedance matching between circuits; (2) **pre-amplifiers,** used to detect and amplify extremely small signals which are then fed into another amplifier; and (3) **null-balance amplifiers,** used in instrument detecting circuits (as a type of amplifying Wheatstone bridge).

AMPLIFIER TYPES BY OPERATING FREQUENCY

Amplifiers are designed to operate over specified frequency ranges, determined, in most cases, by the types and values of the components used in their design. There are three general classes:
1. **Audio amplifiers,** amplifying signals ranging from 15 Hz up to as high as 20,000 Hz.
2. **Video-amplifiers,** similar in design to audio amplifiers, and covering a range of frequencies from 20 Hz to 6M Hz, and sometimes higher.
3. **RF (radio frequency) amplifiers,** narrow band amplifiers operating anywhere within the range of 30,000 Hz to 30M Hz.

A slightly more detailed discussion of some of the above circuits is presented in Chapter 19.

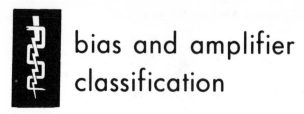# bias and amplifier classification

CHAPTER 10

BIAS

The many terms used to identify various voltages applied to different segments of an amplifier circuit can be confusing to the uninitiated. Before we add yet another term it might be helpful to clarify some previously mentioned terminology:

1. **B+ voltage:**
   This term refers to a relatively high DC voltage usually applied to the plate circuit of an amplifier, or other vacuum tube circuit, sometimes loosely referred to as *power.*

2. **Signal voltages (input signal, output signal or plate signal):**
   These terms are used to refer to the AC voltage appearing at the grid (input signal) and the resulting variations in plate or cathode voltage (output signal).

3. **Filament (heater) voltage:**
   This voltage is the AC voltage (usually 6.3 or 12.6 volts) used to heat the filaments of vacuum tubes.

4. **Bias voltage:**
   Bias voltage is the fixed DC potential on the grid taken with respect to the cathode when no input signal is present. With a signal present at the grid, the grid voltage then becomes the sum of the bias and the signal voltages. (A somewhat different sense is implied in semiconductor circuitry in Chapter 12.)

The bias voltage on the grid of a vacuum tube has much to do with determining how the tube will operate. Selecting the proper value of bias can cause a triode to function as a linear amplifier, a nonlinear amplifier, a power amplifier (when used push-pull), or even as a type of rectifier.

94

TYPES OF BIAS

Bias voltage is chosen by reference to the characteristic curve of the tube in order to produce a particular type of operation. In Figure 10-1, the curve represents a characteristic curve of a triode, showing the plate current values (I_p) for various amounts of grid voltage (E_g) at one fixed value of $B+$. (Other similar curves may be drawn for other values of the $B+$ voltage.) Note that a linear change in I_p occurs only from -10 volts to +15 volts. Below and above these two values, respectively, I_p does not change proportionally with E_g. Choosing a bias such that E_g always remains on the straight line will give undistorted amplification.

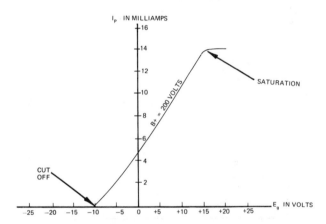

Fig. 10-1: An E_g-I_p characteristic curve showing saturation (I_p=maximum) and cutoff (I_p=zero) with a fixed B+ of 200 volts

As an example, in Figure 10-2 assume we have a bias of +10 volts, and an input signal of 20 volts peak to peak is injected into the grid circuit. As the signal goes 10 volts positive, the grid (E_g) goes positive from +10 to +20. However, at the point when E_g = +15, the tube is at saturation. Above that point, the positive change on the grid causes no further change in I_p, and consequently, the output signal will be distorted (its peak clipped off).

To look at bias in the other direction, assume we have a bias of -5 volts with the same input signal. As the input goes 10 volts positive, I_p increases, then returns to normal since the grid goes from -5 to +5 volts and back to -5 volts. When the input swings 10 volts negative, E_g decreases to a minimum of -15. However, at E_g = -10, no further change in I_p occurs, since the tube is cut off. All the grid signal below -10 volts is lost, resulting in an output signal distortion. (Again, the peak is clipped).

Since E_p varies inversely with E_g, the output signal plate voltage is distorted in its negative swing for the first bias value and distorted in its positive swing in the second case.

From this discussion, it is obvious that for linear (undistorted) amplification, a triode must be biased at a point on the linear portion of its characteristic curve and for maximum possible input signal without distortion on the bias should be at the midpoint of the linear portion of the curve.

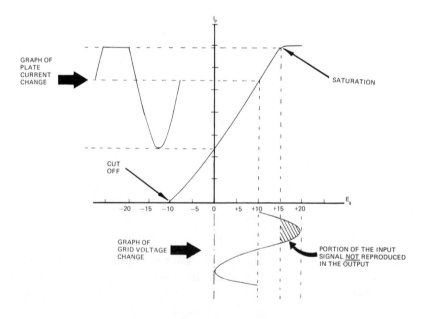

Fig. 10-2: Amplifier distortion

METHODS OF PRODUCING BIAS

There are three methods of producing bias voltage. Two employ components that are part of the amplifier circuitry, and the third produces the bias voltage externally (in another circuit).

Cathode Bias

Cathode bias is developed by making use of the unidirectional current flow through the tube. A resistor (R_K) is inserted in the cathode circuit. With no voltage on the grid $(E_g = 0)$, when current flows through the tube a positive potential is developed on the cathode (Figure 10-3). Since bias refers to the potential of the grid with respect to E_K, the grid is then negative with respect to the cathode.

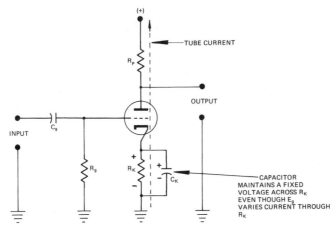

Fig. 10-3: Cathode biasing – with cathode at a positive potential grid becomes negative with respect to cathode

The input signal will tend to cause variations in the current flowing through R_K, the cathode resistor (since it controls current through the whole system). A capacitor (C_K) placed in parallel with the bias resistor is used to keep the bias voltage relatively constant. Such a capacitor is designated a cathode "by-pass" capacitor. It functions by first charging to the bias value across R_K and, as current through R_K varies, charging or discharging through R_K to compensate for the changes.

Grid Leak Bias

At times referred to as **automatic bias,** grid leak bias is developed only when an input signal is present. The input signal draws grid current and charges an RC (resistive-capacitive) network which results in a negative bias on the grid. This is accomplished by the capacitor charging during the first 90° of the input, then discharging (through R), slowly, during the remaining 270°.

Fixed Bias

Fixed bias is produced by an external voltage source, such as a C battery or a tapped DC power supply. A positive voltage can be applied directly to the cathode or a negative voltage to the grid, producing the same bias effect either way.

AMPLIFIER CLASSIFICATION

Amplifiers are operationally classified on two criteria: (1) the point at which they are biased on the characteristic curve and (2) the period (based on input signal time) for which plate current flows.

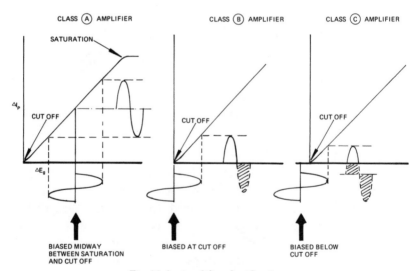

Fig. 10-4: Amplifier classification

1. *Class A* amplifiers are biased midway between saturation and cut-off. Such biasing allows plate current to flow and an output to be produced during 360° of the input.

2. *Class B* amplifiers are biased at cut-off, allowing plate current to flow for 180° of the input.

3. *Class C* amplifiers are biased below cut-off. Plate current flows for less than 180° of the input.

Figure 10-4 shows the relationship of E_g to I_p in each of these classes of amplifiers.

Although a Class A amplifier normally allows I_p to flow for 360° of the input, this condition is not obtained if the input signal is of such magnitude that it drives the grid beyond both saturation and cut-off. This condition, known as "over-driving" the amplifier, is normally undesirable; however, it can sometimes be used selectively to "clip" undesirable peaks from a signal.

AMPLIFIER COUPLING METHODS

Most signals found in biomedical instrumentation require a great deal of amplification. In order to accomplish this, more than one stage of amplification is required; therefore, circuits are needed to couple the stages together. Two or more amplifier stages coupled together are generally referred to as a *cascade*. There are three methods commonly used to accomplish this: (1) **direct coupling**, (2) **resistive-capacitive**—or **RC-coupling**, and (3) **transformer coupling**.

Direct coupling is used only with extremely stable or chopper type amplifier systems, and involves directly connecting the output of one circuit to the input of the next.

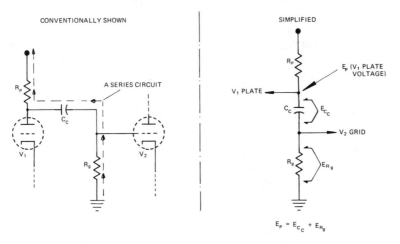

Fig. 10-5: Resistive-capacitive (RC) coupling

RC coupling is widely used in both tube and transistor type circuits. A capacitor is hooked from the output of the first stage by way of a resistor to ground; the input of the next stage is hooked between the two. Since the capacitor is actually in parallel with the first stage, any fluctuations across the stage are followed by the capacitor, charging and discharging through the resistor. These fluctuations are felt at the input to the next stage, since it is hooked across the resistor. The capacitor, since all capacitors show high impedance to DC, blocks the DC voltage of the first stage (the normally high plate or collector potential) from appearing at the input of the next stage. RC coupling can be summarized by noting that (1) it blocks DC, but (2) passes the AC signal.

Transformer coupling is used in circuit applications that require either (1) isolation, (2) impedance matching, or (3) high selectivity. The output of the first stage is attached to the primary coil of a coupling transformer and the input of the second stage to the transformer's secondary winding. The signal is transferred by conventional transformer action from the primary to the secondary coil of the transformer. With appropriate capacitances added, coupling transformers can also function as resonant filters, passing only predetermined signal frequencies, which make them highly selective devices.

DISTORTION IN AMPLIFIERS

Distortion of a signal that is being processed by an amplifier can be due to various causes, but the two factors most often encountered are:

1. *Over-driving the amplifier:* This results in one, or both, peaks of the output signal being "clipped."

2. *Poor amplifier frequency response:* The frequency response of an amplifier can be divided into two areas: high and low. The effects of poor low frequency response are most often due to the *RC* coupling used, while poor high frequency response is generally caused by stray (inter-electrode) capacitance.

The frequency response of an amplifier can be best evaluated by injecting a square wave signal and observing the resulting output signal. This is because a square wave contains both high and low frequency components, and amplifier distortion manifests itself by producing characteristic changes in the square wave. Low frequency distortion alters the flat (horizontal) portion of a square wave, which represents the low frequency components, while high frequency distortion alters the vertical portion of the wave, which contains the high frequency components. The effects of poor response in each of these areas are shown in Figure 10-6. Methods that have been developed to compensate for the effects of poor frequency response include the use of (1) *selective compensating networks* and (2) *degenerative (negative) feedback.* A parallel *RC* network in series with an amplifier plate (or collector) load resistor will compensate selectively for low frequency distortion, or an increase in the values of the RC coupling components can accomplish the same result. The latter method is not often used since it tends to adversely affect the high frequency response of the circuit. Selective compensation for high frequency distortion may be obtained by adding an *RF* "peaking coil" in series with the amplifier's plate (or collector) load resistor, using a pentode tube, or decreasing the size of the plate (collector) load resistor. The latter method can have an adverse effect on low frequency response and cause decreased gain.

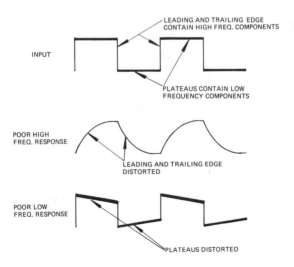

Fig. 10-6: Effect of poor amplifier frequency response to a square wave input signal

The use of degenerative or negative feedback will compensate for poor response at both the low and high ends of the amplifier's operating spectrum; it also, however, causes decreased gain. Even with this drawback, degenerative feedback compensation is the method of choice in most circuit applications. Two techniques often used to accomplish this are (1) using an output to grid (input) coupling resistor to feed back a portion of the output signal to the input, or (2) eliminating the cathode (or emitter) bypass capacitor usually found in an amplifier circuit. Both methods produce the same general effect, decreased distortion and decreased gain. The overall sequential action of one kind of feed-back compensation is shown in Figure 10-7.

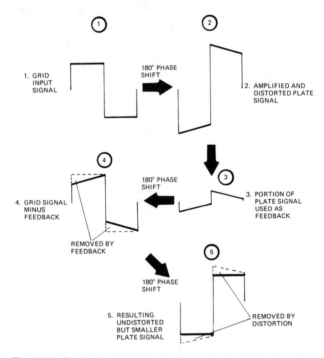

Fig. 10-7: Feedback compensation for low frequency distortion

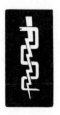

special purpose tubes

CHAPTER 11

INTERELECTRODE CAPACITANCE

Any two metallic conductors separated by a dielectric form a capacitor. Since a triode vacuum tube consists of three such metallic conductors (plate, grid, and cathode), and these are in turn separated by a dielectric (a vacuum), the conditions required for capacitive action exist. The capacitance present between any two elements of a triode is called **interelectrode capacitance**, and

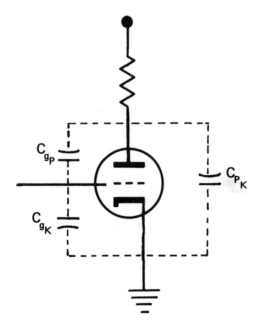

Fig. 11-1: *Schematic representation of interelectrode capacitance. Adapted from Air Force Manual 52-8, Electronic Circuit Analysis-modified by the author. (courtesy of the United States Air Force)*

three separate interelectrode capacitances are present: grid-to-plate (C_{gp}), grid-to-cathode (C_{gk}), and plate to cathode (C_{pk}). Figure 11-1 is a schematic representation. The interelectrode capacitance having the greatest effect on the triode operation is C_{gp}. This capacitance offers a path by which variations in plate voltage can be fed back to the grid input circuit: a process known as **feedback**. Because of the frequency dependence of capacitive reactance, feedback is negligible at low (audio) frequencies and increases at higher frequencies. It is obvious that interelectrode capacitance can produce undesirable effects in amplifiers at high frequencies by coupling back a portion of the plate signal to the grid, thereby distorting the grid signal. The higher the frequency, the greater the effect of interelectrode capacitance, and the greater the amount of distortion produced. This undesirable effect limits the upper frequencies at which triodes can function as distortionless amplifiers and resulted in the development of the *tetrode* vacuum tube. Tetrodes are capable of amplifying without distortion at frequencies above the limit of triode amplifiers.

TETRODES

A **tetrode** is a tube having *four* elements: cathode, control grid, screen grid, and plate. The screen grid is placed between the grid and the plate; it reduces the effects of plate-to-grid interelectrode capacitance and minimizes feedback. A capacitor called a *screen by-pass* (C_{Sg}) capacitor is connected from the screen grid to

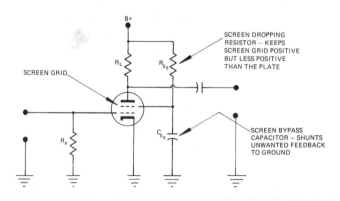

Fig. 11-2: A tetrode amplifier

ground. Feedback effects which would ordinarily reach the input circuit are passed to ground through this capacitor and their undesirable action on the input avoided. Figure 11-2 is a schematic diagram of a tetrode. Note the "screen by-pass" capacitor (C_{Sg}).

PENTODES

The screen grid in a tetrode, since it is operated at a high positive potential (though not quite as high as the plate), accelerates electrons passing to the plate. Upon striking the plate, these high velocity electrons cause secondary emission. Secondarily emitted electrons travel toward the electrode exerting the greatest influence on them. At high plate voltages, this poses no problem. However, when the plate swings to its low value, the screen grid begins to draw this secondary current. To eliminate excess screen grid current, a third grid is added called a **suppressor** grid. Placed between the plate and the screen grid and connected to the cathode, the suppressor grid repels secondary emitted electrons back toward the plate. It has negligible effect on primary electrons from the cathode, since primary electrons are accelerated by the screen grid and are of a much higher kinetic energy level than secondary electrons.

The pentode has virtually replaced the tetrode as an amplifier in most circuit applications. However, special tetrodes known as **beam power tubes,** are used as high power amplifiers. Figure 11-3 shows a schematic diagram of a pentode.

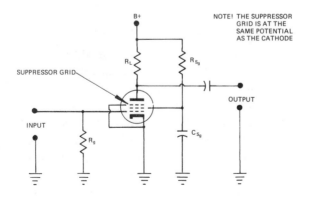

Fig. 11-3: A pentode amplifier

BEAM POWER TUBES

The construction of a beam power amplifier differs from that of normal voltage amplifiers in the following ways: (1) larger and more rugged electrodes, (2) designed to dissipate heat, (3) grid-wire spacing increased (to allow more current), and (4) greater emitting ability built into cathode.

The beam power tube, generally considered a tetrode, has the characteristics of a pentode due to its unusual design. The density of the electron beam to the plate is so great it prevents secondary emission. Beam forming plates (a type of screen grid) connected to the cathode concentrate the electron stream even more before it strikes the plate. In Figure 11-4 schematics of typical beam power tetrodes are shown. Note the beam forming plates.

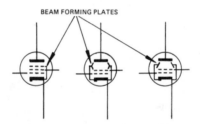

Fig. 11-4: Beam power tubes - technically pentodes since they have five elements. Reproduced from Air Force Manual 52-8, Electronic Circuit Analysis. (courtesy of the United States Air Force)

REMOTE CUT-OFF TUBES

The grid wiring in most tubes is uniformly spaced so that when the bias is such that it is able to stop current through one part of the grid, it stops current through all of the grid. Such grids are called *sharp cut-off grids*. The grid wiring in a *remote cut-off tube* is not uniform; consequently current is stopped in a more gradual way (Figure 11-5). In such a tube, when bias is made to vary with the strength of the input signal, it causes the stronger signals to be amplified less than the weaker signals yielding a more constant output. Such applications are found in automatic gain control (AGC) circuits or automatic volume control (AVC) circuits.

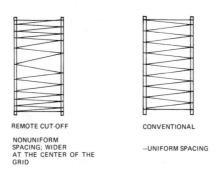

REMOTE CUT-OFF

NONUNIFORM
SPACING; WIDER
AT THE CENTER OF THE
GRID

CONVENTIONAL

—UNIFORM SPACING

Fig. 11-5: Comparison of conventional grid wiring with remote cut-off wiring

GAS-FILLED TUBES

Gas-filled tubes will be considered along with vacuum tubes, although in the strict sense of the word they are not "vacuum" tubes. Gas-filled tubes are evacuated and then filled with low pressure gas—usually nitrogen, neon, argon, or mercury vapor.

Gas-filled tubes can be classified as either hot or cold cathode tubes, depending upon whether or not a filament is used to heat the cathode.

Normally gasses are poor conductors. However, when ionized, they become good conductors, and it is in this way that gas tubes are utilized. In the *cold cathode* gas tube a specific value of voltage must be impressed across the tube to produce ionization. In the *hot cathode* gas tube, electrons emitted by the cathode and drawn to the positive plate produce ionization upon striking the gas molecules in the tube. The unique characteristic of gas tubes is that once the tube is ionized, *the potential across the tube remains nearly constant—even though the current through the tube may vary.* This is accomplished as follows: As the current through the tube increases, ionization increases. However, as ionization *increases,* the tube resistance *decreases.* Therefore, the voltage drop across the tube ($E = I \times R$) remains relatively constant. This characteristic makes cold cathode gas tubes useful as power supply voltage regulators. Load current can vary within specified limits, yet the voltage supplied by the tube remains constant.

In power supplies which produce large rectified currents, regular diode vacuum tubes are replaced by hot cathode gas tubes, the most popular being the mercury-vapor tube. Such tubes are capable of handling 100 amperes or more while high vacuum diodes are limited to currents below one ampere.

THYRATRONS

A hot cathode gas tube with a control grid is known as a **thyratron**. The bias on the grid is used *only* to determine the value of the plate voltage required to produce ionization. Once the tube ionizes, the grid is no longer effective, the tube acting as a diode. The control grid does not regain control until the tube deionizes. Such tubes are often used as sawtooth wave generators and in various types of control circuits. Figure 11-6 shows schematic diagrams of various types of gas tubes.

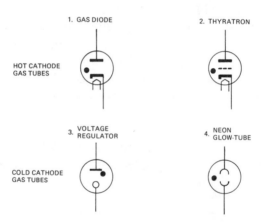

Fig. 11-6: Schematic representations of gas filled tubes. Reproduced from Air Force Manual 52-8, Electronic Circuit Analysis. (courtesy of the United States Air Force)

CATHODE RAY TUBES (CRT)

The **cathode ray tube** (CRT) is a specialized type of vacuum tube in which the electrons emitted from the cathode are formed into a narrow beam and projected onto a phosphor-coated screen. Upon striking the screen, the electron beams cause it to glow at the point of impact. The beam can be controlled to move horizontally or vertically, causing the glowing spot at the point of contact to move.

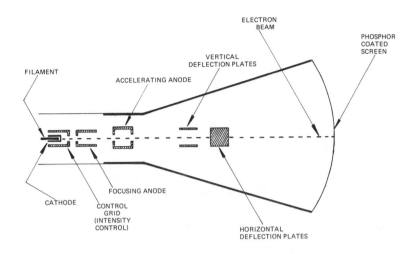

Fig. 11-7: A simplified diagram of a cathode ray tube (CRT)

Figure 11-7 is a simplified schematic of a CRT. The *electron gun* consists of the heater, cathode, grid, first (focusing) anode, and second (accelerating) anode. A focused, narrow beam of electrons is ejected from the electron gun, and projected onto the screen. With no signal voltages applied to the deflection plates, an adjustable DC voltage on the plates enables the spot to be centered. After the spot is centered, two signal voltages must be injected to produce a wave pattern on the screen. The first is the **sweep voltage.** When this signal is applied repeatedly to the *horizontal* deflection plates it causes the spot to move across the screen horizontally from left to right and then to jump back quickly and repeat this motion. Figure 11-8(*A*) shows the applied wave form and the trace it produces on the face of the CRT. The second signal injected is the unknown or *test signal* which is to be viewed and analyzed. This voltage is applied to the *vertical* deflection plates, causing the beam to be deflected up or down at the same time the sweep voltage is moving the beam horizontally. Figure 11-8(*B*) shows the result of the simultaneous application of these inputs. Note that the frequency of an unknown voltage can be determined by injecting it as a vertical signal along with a horizontal signal of known frequency.

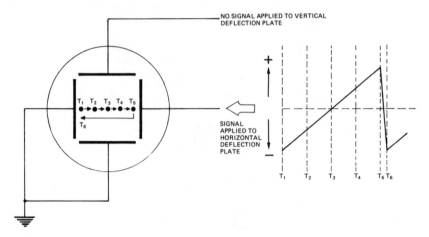

Fig. 11-8(A): Result of applying a sawtooth signal to the horizontal deflection plates of a CRT

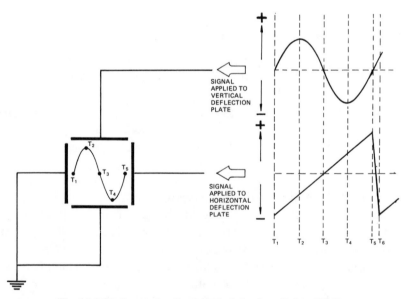

Fig. 11-8(B): Sweep signal and vertical signal applied to C.R.T.

Example: If the horizontal sweep frequency is 1,000 cps and an unknown vertical input shows one cycle on the screen, then its frequency must also be 1,000 cps. If the unknown input shows two cycles on the screen (it goes through two cycles while the sweep signal goes through one), its frequency is 2,000 cps.

PHOTO-TUBES

Photo-tubes are vacuum or gas-filled electron tubes containing two elements: (1) a curved photosensitive cathode, and (2) a positively charged anode.

When radiant energy strikes the cathode, electrons—called **photo-electrons**—are emitted from its surface. These negative particles are attracted by the positive anode and the result is a current flow in the external circuit. Since the number of photo-electrons emitted by the cathode is proportional to the amount of radiant energy striking it, the photo-current produced is a direct measure of light intensity.

There is little variation between vacuum and gas photo-diodes in general construction. The major difference is that the latter contain an inert gas such as argon which ionizes when struck with sufficient energy by photo-electrons. This ionization results in a somewhat amplified photo-current. Consequently, gas photo-diodes are used when we need to detect lower levels of illumination. Figure 11-9 shows a typical photo-diode.

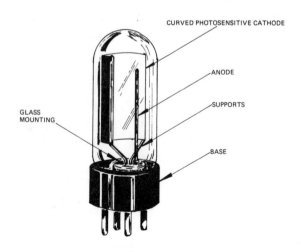

Fig. 17-11: A simplified phototube (photodiode)

When very low levels of light or minute variations in intensity are involved, photo-multipliers are used in place of photo-diodes (Figure 11-10).

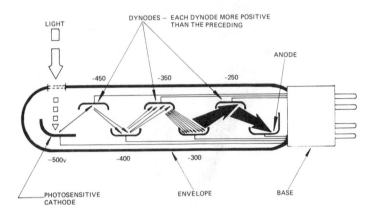

Fig. 11-10: Pictorial diagram of a typical photomultiplier

Photo-multipliers consist of a *photo-cathode,* a series of special electrodes called *dynodes,* and a *positive anode.* Each dynode is sequentially at a more positive potential than the preceding one.

When light causes a photo-electron to be emitted from the cathode, the photo-electron is drawn to the first dynode. When it strikes the dynode, more electrons are ejected from the surface of the dynode due to secondary emission (*cf* Chapter 8).

These secondary electrons (as they are called) are focused by way of baffles to the next dynode where the action is again repeated, and this process continues until the electron stream reaches the anode. External circuit current then results.

Since the action of an electron striking each dynode results in multiple secondary electrons being emitted, the factor of amplification or gain in this type tube can be as great as 1,000,000.

STORAGE CATHODE RAY TUBES

A limitation common to the conventional cathode ray tube (CRT) is the rapid loss of image luminescence, especially when the tube is used to monitor slow frequency signals. In other words, as an electron beam is moved slowly across the face of a cathode ray tube, the image it produces tends to fade rapidly. Within the last decade, significant improvements in CRT design technology have solved this problem; today, oscilloscopes are available with CRT's capable of storing a single event (image) for up to an hour. Using special CRT's and control circuitry, these **storage oscilloscopes**, as they are called, provide capability for storing, erasing, and, in some cases, enhancing images on their screens. The one drawback of these oscilloscopes is their expense. The specialized CRT's and control circuitry required in their manufacture make expensive oscilloscopes even more expensive, and therefore impractical for some users. Recent advances in engineering design have provided storage capabilities in oscilloscopes which use a conventional CRT. However, these developments have not yet filtered down to the routine oscilloscope marketplace and such scopes are not widely available.

A typical storage oscilloscope functions on the same basic principles as a conventional oscilloscope, but with a few very important design differences incorporated into its structure. A conventional scope contains a cathode ray tube with a single electron beam which is "fired" from an electron gun at a phosphorescent screen (coating on the face of the tube) to produce a visual image. As the beam is deflected horizontally or vertically across the tube's face to produce the monitored image, the trace remains for a few seconds, then disappears. In contrast, the cathode ray tube in a storage oscilloscope has *two electron guns* which function as follows:

One gun (the **writing gun**) fires a narrow, high energy, focused writing beam at the screen. The other gun (the **flood gun**) fires a wide, blanket, or dispersed low energy beam which covers the whole screen. Immediately in front of the screen (between the electron guns and the screen itself) is a special dielectric material held at a negative potential. In some cases the dielectric is a mesh; in others it is a coating of scattered particles. The high energy beam can easily penetrate the dielectric to produce an image on the tube's face. The low energy beam, however, cannot penetrate the dielectric (due to its negative charge) and therefore does *not* strike the screen or produce an image. Now, how does this tube store an image? Let us see.

When the writing beam is off, no image is seen on the tube's face. As soon as the writing beam is triggered, its high energy electron beam strikes the dielectric. The high energy particles cause a change of state (negative to positive) in the charge on the dielectric at the point of impact, as a result of secondary electron emission (Chapter 8). Once this is accomplished, and the writing beam is removed, the low energy flood beam is allowed to penetrate the dielectric at the point of impact, strike the screen, and maintain the image. As long as the dielectric is kept in the positively charged condition, the image is held on the screen by the flood beam; it is "stored." When required, additional circuitry can be activated to return the dielectric to its original negative state, blocking the flood beam and "erasing" the image from the screen.

As noted previously, storage oscilloscopes are ideal for monitoring slowly generated physiological signals such as ECG's and EEG's. However, until recently the expense of storage cathode ray tubes and the associated circuitry required priced them out of the medical electronics market. Recent engineering and design developments have made some inroads into this area and one company, Mennen-Greatbatch Electronics of Clarence, New York, manufacturers of clinical monitoring systems, utilize integrated and semiconductor computer type circuitry to provide image persistence without resorting to expensive storage cathode ray tubes. The Mennen-Greatbatch technique, called **non-fade memory** employs MOS shift register memory circuits and analog to digital conversion of the ECG signal to constantly refresh the image on a low persistence phosphor screen. The image is refreshed at a high rate which compensates for the low persistence of the phosphor. The memory is nonsynchronous in nature; in other words, it continually slips, allowing a new bit of information to be stored as another is dropped (as in a car wash, as one car enters, one exits). In this way as one element of a signal begins to pass off the tube, the next is ready for viewing. This new innovation should prove to be advantageous and eagerly welcomed by nurses in hospital intensive care units who are often required to monitor multiple traces which appear and disappear on the screen at frustratingly odd and unsynchronized intervals.

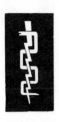

semiconductor fundamentals

CHAPTER 12

In the discussion of the theory of current flow through a conductor (considering the transit time during which an electron is passing from one atom to the next), we were introduced to the concept of an *"electron-hole" charge pair* consisting of (a) a transient electron, and (b) an electron-hole (the position which the electron had vacated). When electron current flows in the direction from a negative potential toward a more positive potential, there occurs at the same time what appears to be a relative migration of positive charges in the opposite direction. Positive charge migration, termed **hole current**, is important in the theory of semiconductors. In some materials, the number of free electrons and the number of apparent holes are not the same. One or the other is in excess.

When current flows through a material containing many free electrons, negative charges (electrons) represent the majority charge-carrying elements. In a material with an excess of holes (*i.e.,* there are bond gaps in its crystal structure) the majority charge-carrying elements are the holes. (For example: when current passes through a conductor containing an excess of holes, it appears (at any single instant in time) that there are more holes than electrons in motion). By combining two such substances, each with different charge-carrying elements—one with holes, the other with electrons—semiconductor devices are made. Semiconductors have virtually replaced vacuum tubes in most electronic circuit applications because of their desirable characteristics of (1) low power requirements, (2) reliability, (3) compactness, and (4) longer life. Before continuing further we should examine briefly just how semiconductors are made.

DONOR AND ACCEPTOR MATERIALS

Pure semiconductor materials are not really semiconductors; they are practically insulators. It is the addition of "extra" electrons or holes to a pure semiconductor substance that transforms it into an active current-carrying element. Let us take germanium as an example and see how this is accomplished.

A germanium atom has four electrons in its outer shell, in which the maximum number possible is 32. In a germanium crystal, the outer shell electrons of each atom form covalent bonds with neighbor atoms. This arrangement is very stable and no electrons are free for current flow; consequently, intrinsic (pure) germanium is considered an insulator.

The addition of a small amount of a properly selected impurity changes the conductivity of germanium. The impurities create either an excess or a deficiency of electrons. The chemical properties of the impurities are such that their atoms form covalent bonds with the germanium atoms and fit easily into the crystal structure. However, if the added material has *one electron too many* per atom, these extra electrons are not covalently bound and are available to carry current. Such an added impurity is called a **pentavalent** or **donor impurity**. Should the substance added, however, contain *one electron too few* per atom, each atom will attempt to borrow an electron from its neighbor, thereby creating a hole or electron deficiency in the crystal. This type of material is known as a **trivalent** or **acceptor impurity**. Some typical impurities used in semiconductor manufacturing include:

Trivalent or Acceptor Impurities	Pentavalent or Donor Impurities
Aluminum	Arsenic
Gallium	Antimony
Indium	Bismuth
Boron	Phosphorus

Semiconductor crystals with excess electrons (donor impurity) are known as **negative carriers** or *N*-type materials. Crystals with excess holes (acceptor impurity) are known as **positive carriers** or *P*-type materials.

N-TYPE AND P-TYPE CURRENT FLOW

Application of a voltage across an *N*-type semiconductor causes current flow due to negative carriers (electrons) as shown in Figure 12-1. This follows the pattern of, and can be envisioned as, electron current in a normal metallic conductor.

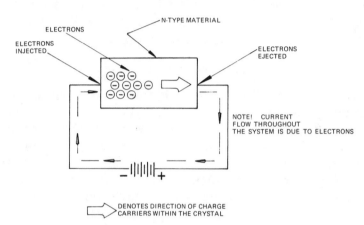

Fig. 12-1: Current flow through N-type semiconductor material

Application of a voltage across a *P*-type semiconductor also causes current to flow, but in a somewhat different manner. In Figure 12-2 the *P*-type material has an excess of holes; electrons flowing from the negative battery terminal "cancel" holes at the

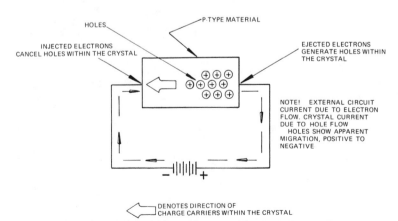

Fig. 12-2: Current flow through P-type semiconductor material

crystal-wire interface on the left. At the other end of the crystal, electrons (attracted to the positive charge) "generate" holes as they leave the crystal and pass into the wire. These new holes show apparent movement toward the negative side of the crystal while electrons move in the opposite direction. The actions of hole cancellations and hole generation occur simultaneously, thus maintaining the charge equilibrium of the crystal. Figure 2-1, Chapter 2, is another example of this process.

P-N JUNCTION DIODES

Before studying *P-N* junctions, it must be emphasized that the addition of impurity atoms to a semiconductor material during the manufacturing process does *not* give the material a net charge imbalance. The crystal remains neutral since all electron charges added are balanced by the proton charges added along with them. The "excess" electrons are just easier to excite into a current-carrying state, since they are "loose" within the crystal structure. In the case of the excess positive charges, the holes make it easier to move electrons normally covalently bound, (with covalent bonding the electrons have no extra holes to move into).

By chemically fusing a *P*-type and an *N*-type crystal together, a *P-N* junction is formed. At the interface between the two materials, a process called **carrier diffusion** occurs, resulting in

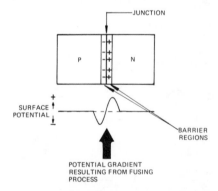

Fig. 12-3: Surface potential measured along a crystal made of a segment of P-type semiconductor fused to a segment of N-type semiconductor

some electrons passing into the *P*-type material. However, as soon as these electrons pass over the junction, the electrically neutral state of each crystal is disturbed and two permanently charged areas called **barrier regions** result. The electrons form a *negative* charge barrier in the *P*-type material while the holes (generated in the *N*-type by the electrons that have left) form a *positive* charge barrier in the *N*-type material. The **potential gradient** produced by these barrier regions prevents any further charge movement. The distribution of potential across the surface of such a semiconductor junction is shown in the graph in Figure 12-3.

Before current can be made to flow across a *P-N* junction, the potential gradient must first be overcome by an external energy source that gives the charges enough energy to pass through the barrier regions and across the junction. Such external energy sources are referred to as **biases.**

FORWARD AND REVERSE BIAS

In Figure 12-4 (A), the positive lead of the battery is connected to the *P*-type material and the negative lead to the *N*-type. This type of polarization across a junction is known as **forward bias.** The positively charged holes are forced toward the junction by the positive terminal, while electrons are repelled toward the junction by the negative terminal. Holes and electrons pass into the barrier region where they recombine, eliminating charge pairs. Simultaneously new charge pairs are generated due to (1) injection of electrons into *N*-type material from the battery negative lead, and

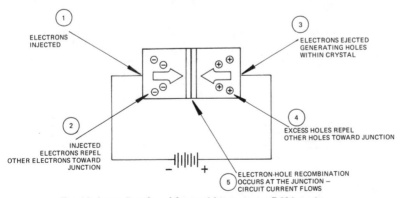

Fig. 12-4(A): Results of forward bias across a P-N junction

(2) generation of holes in the *P*-type material due to ejection of electrons into the wire toward the positive terminal. The net result is current flow from the battery negative terminal through the *P-N* junction to the positive terminal. The amount of current flow is determined by the number of electron hole recombinations that occur in the barrier region which in turn is indirectly determined by the amount of bias voltage applied.

In Figure 12-4 (*B*) the battery is reversed: negative lead to *P*-type positive lead to *N*-type. This polarization of the junction is known as **reverse bias**. The holes now tend to be attracted to the negative charge area and the electrons to the positive charge area, both moving away from the junction; the result is no recombination in the barrier region and consequently no current flow. What actually happens is that the potential gradient is effectively made larger by the reverse bias. The effects of bias voltages across a *P-N* junction can be summarized as follows:

A. *Forward bias:* positive to *P*-type material, negative to *N*-type material. Any increase in forward bias tends to increase current flow through the junction.

B. *Reverse bias:* positive to *N*-type material, negative to *P*-type material. Any increase in reverse bias tends to decrease current flow through the junction.

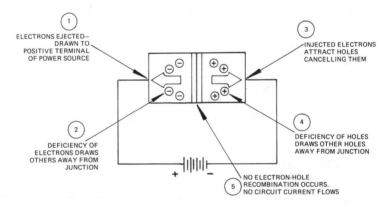

ELECTRONS EJECTED—
DRAWN TO
POSITIVE TERMINAL
OF POWER SOURCE

INJECTED ELECTRONS
ATTRACT HOLES
CANCELLING THEM

DEFICIENCY OF
ELECTRONS DRAWS
OTHERS AWAY FROM
JUNCTION

DEFICIENCY OF HOLES
DRAWS OTHER HOLES
AWAY FROM JUNCTION

NO ELECTRON-HOLE
RECOMBINATION OCCURS.
NO CIRCUIT CURRENT FLOWS

Fig. 12-4(B): Results of reverse bias across a P-N junction.

This summary applies to any semiconductor junction. Remembering this capsule of information will very much simplify the study of semiconductor devices.

JUNCTION DIODE—APPLICATION

From the discussion of forward and reverse bias it becomes clear that the P-N junction is a unidirectional current device—just like a vacuum tube. Therefore, such a junction can be used as a rectifier. The diagram in Figure 12-5 shows a P-N junction functioning as a half-wave rectifier. On the first half cycle of the input, the junction is *forward biased* and forward current flows in the circuit. On the second half cycle, the polarity of the voltage has reversed and the junction is *reverse biased*. It is at this point that a difference between semiconductor diodes and vacuum tube diodes becomes apparent. With reverse polarity across a vacuum tube diode, the tube will not normally conduct, (*i.e.*, no current will flow from plate to cathode). However, with a semiconductor diode, a small amount of reverse current flows when the junction is reverse biased. This reverse current is due to the **minority charge carriers** (electrons in P-type, holes in N-type). The result is a small negative dip of the output signal as shown in Figure 12-5. Normally the small amount of reverse current flowing through a junction will not cause damage; however, should the bias voltage reach a high enough value, reverse current can

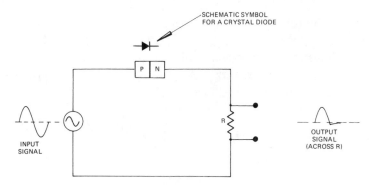

Fig. 12-5: A P-N junction functioning as a rectifier. On the first half cycle the crystal is forward biased; therefore, it conducts. On the second half cycle the junction is reverse biased and only a slight reverse current flows (minority carrier current)

suddenly increase dramatically (due to electrons being pulled from valence bonds), giving way at the reverse breakdown point to a phenomenon called **avalanche current**. When this occurs in a conventional semiconductor diode, it destroys the integrity of the junction, ruining it. Some specially designed semiconductor diodes, however, function at their reverse breakdown point, utilizing avalanche current. These diodes are called **Zener diodes** and find applications as voltage regulators (*cf* Chapter 16).

Figure 12-6 shows current-voltage curves for both a junction diode and a Zener diode. Note that the reverse breakdown point of a normal diode is called the *Zener point* in the Zener diode.

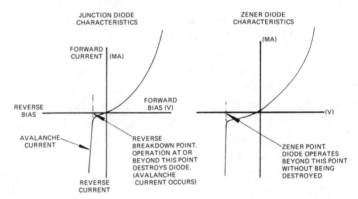

Fig. 12-6:   Comparison of characteristic curve of a junction diode with that of a
              Zener diode

Semiconductor diodes can replace vacuum tube diodes in almost all applications except those involving very high current values. No doubt as the science of electronic materials progresses, semiconductor replacements will eventually be found for every type of vacuum tube.

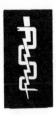

transistor amplifiers

CHAPTER 13

TRANSISTOR FUNDAMENTALS

The beginning of solid state electronics can be traced back to the days of crystal radio sets for these devices employed a point contact crystal diode as a rectifier. This type of diode was made by attaching a catswhisker wire to a germanium crystal (Figure 13-1). A diode constructed in this way shows a high resistance to current in one direction and a low resistance in the opposite direction; consequently it is able to function as a unidirectional current device. This same basic design concept is used in many miniature crystal diodes today. Although after development of the triode crystal radio sets were soon supplanted by vacuum tube units, the history of solid-state point contact devices made full circle in 1948 with the development of the **point contact transistor.** If we attach two metal catswhiskers close together on the surface of a small wafer of *P* or *N* type semiconductor material, and pass a relatively high current through the catswhiskers and crystal, the areas around each point of contact become opposite in charge structure to the original crystal (*e.g.,* they

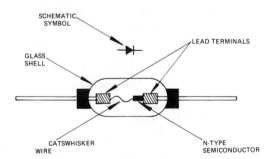

Fig. 13-1: Pictorial diagram of a point contact diode

123

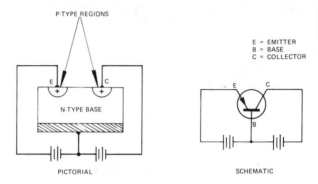

Fig. 13-2: A point contact transistor

become *P*-type if the original material was *N*-type). The result is a three element semiconductor device, the **transistor**. Figure 13-2 shows pictorial and schematic diagrams of a point contact transistor. The transistor is capable of performing most of the operations that are accomplished by vacuum tubes and consequently, due to its many advantages, has virtually replaced the vacuum tube except in a few special applications.

Today, the **junction transistor** has, for economic reasons, replaced the point contact transistor since the latter is the more difficult of the two to manufacture. However, the basic theory behind the operation of these devices is similar, and an examination of the operation of junction transistors will also encompass the essentials of point contact transistor theory.

THE JUNCTION TRANSISTOR

A junction transistor consists of two *P*-type or two *N*-type germanium or silicon crystals with a crystal wafer of the opposite type sandwiched between them. The result is either a *PNP* or an *NPN* junction transistor. The middle wafer is about 1/10,000 of an inch thick and is called the *base*. The other two elements are the *emitter* and the *collector*. The base is equivalent to the grid of a vacuum tube, while the emitter acts like a cathode and the collector functions like the plate of a tube. In schematic diagrams, the emitter appears as an arrow. It is easy to recognize *PNP* or *NPN* units in a schematic diagram if one remembers the following rule: In a *PNP* schematic symbol, the emitter arrow points to the base—while in a *NPN* diagram the emitter arrow does *not* point to the base (points = *PNP*, not points = *NPN*).

The direction or polarity of a bias voltage at any *PN* junction is considered *forward* if the positive voltage is connected to the *P*-type material and the negative voltage is connected to the *N*-type material. If the connections are the other way (positive (+) to *N*-type and negative (-) to *P*-type), the bias is called *reverse*.

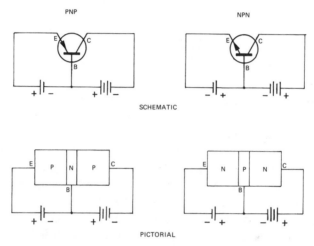

Fig. 13-3: PNP and NPN transistor biasing

Figure 13-3 shows a *PNP* and an *NPN* transistor, each with standard fixed bias. For both transistors, the *emitter-base* junctions are *forward* biased and the *base-collector* junctions are *reverse* biased. When an external signal is applied, it is in the form of a varying voltage connected to one of the transistor leads (usually base or emitter), and the resulting changes in the junction biases cause variations in current flow.

THIS CONFIGURATION OF EMITTER-BASE JUNCTION FORWARD BIASED AND BASE-COLLECTOR JUNCTION REVERSE BIASED IS THE STANDARD FIXED BIAS FORM USED IN ALL JUNCTION TRANSISTOR AMPLIFIERS.

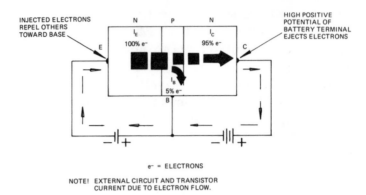

e⁻ = ELECTRONS

NOTE! EXTERNAL CIRCUIT AND TRANSISTOR
CURRENT DUE TO ELECTRON FLOW.

Fig. 13-4: Current flow through an NPN transistor

The operational theory behind fixed bias current through a junction transistor can be seen in Figure 13-4 which shows an *NPN* transistor. A negative potential at the emitter (E) repels electrons toward the base (B) with enough energy to overcome the potential gradient, thereby injecting them into the base region, resulting in emitter to base current (I_B). However, the majority of the electrons from the emitter pass on into the collector (C) for two reasons: (1) the extreme thinness of the base, and (2) the high positive potential at the collector. (Notice that this high positive voltage is the *sum* of *both* bias batteries when taken with reference to the emitter). Since electrons leaving the emitter are directly controlled by the emitter-base bias, emitter current actually *controls* collector current. (In a vacuum tube the parallel situation is control of plate current by bias between grid and cathode.)

Since collector current (I_C) is dependent upon emitter current (I_E) and the value of I_E in turn is dependent upon emitter-base bias, any change in potential at *either* the emitter or the base will vary both I_E and I_C. This characteristic is employed in making the transistor function as an amplifier.

It is important to remember that, in a junction transistor, collector current (I_C) is always less than emitter current (I_E), while base current (I_B) is always less than either of the other two and electrons are the **majority charge carriers.**

The foregoing discussion of current flow through a transistor dealt with an *NPN* device. *PNP* transistor analysis is only slightly

different. Construction of a *PNP* transistor involves combining an
N-type wafer as the base with a *P*-type emitter and collector. To
promote current flow through the transistor requires the appropriate forward and reverse junction biases. (The configuration for
PNP fixed bias is shown in Figure 13-3). The **majority charge
carriers** in PNP transistors are "holes" and the resulting action of
current flow is the same as that described for the *NPN* transistor
except that holes replace electrons.

> *NOTE: To facilitate an understanding of* PNP *devices, the
> reader should try to envision "holes" not just as the
> absence of negative charges in an atom created by
> electron deficiency, but as actual positive charge entities
> (like electrons but with the opposite charge). In
> addition, remember that, whenever a charge pair come
> together and are neutralized, to maintain charge equilib-
> rium within the crystal another pair must be generated.*

Figure 13-5 is an analysis of *PNP* current flow. Positive
bias at the emitter (*E*) repels holes toward the base with enough
energy to overcome the potential gradient and pass on into the
base (*B*) region. Once again, because the base is very thin, and
because of its high (negative) potential, the greater percentage of
"holes" are passed on into the collector (*C*) region where they
recombine with electrons at the *collector-wire* interface. The
overall controlling factor is still the *emitter-base bias* and the
relative current magnitudes of I_B, I_E and I_C are the same as in the
NPN circuit.

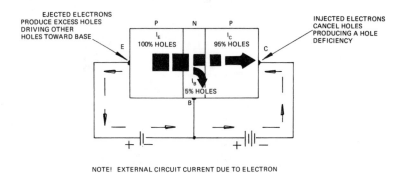

Fig. 13-5: Current flow through a PNP transistor

At this point we again emphasize that in a *NPN* transistor the majority charge carriers are electrons while in a *PNP* transistor the majority charge carriers are "holes."

Although either one of these transistors (*NPN* or *PNP*) can be used in a typical amplifier circuit, the frequency at which the circuit operates is sometimes critical. This is due to the difference in transit time required for the charge pattern to be carried from emitter to collector between *PNP* and *NPN* devices. The mobility of electrons is about twice that of holes. Therefore, a junction transistor with electrons as majority carriers (*NPN*) will have a better frequency response than one employing hole carriers (*PNP*). This fact results in *NPN* transistors generally being used in high frequency amplifier circuits, while *PNP* transistors are used in audio frequency or general purposer amplifier circuitry.

TRANSISTOR AMPLIFIER TYPES

Circuits employing transistors for amplification purposes are divided into three major classes, depending on which element (emitter, base, or collector) is made common to both the input and output circuit, and usually grounded. The three classifications are (1) **common base** circuits, (2) **common emitter** circuits and (3) **common collector** circuits. Typical schematic diagrams for the three types are given in Figure 13-6.

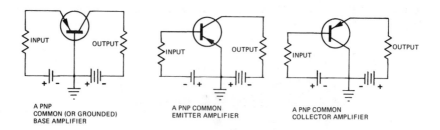

Fig. 13-6: Transistor amplifier configurations

Let us examine the operation of a *PNP* **common base amplifier.** In this circuit the signal voltage is applied *emitter to base* and extracted *collector to base,* with the base grounded (Figure 13-7). By varying the emitter-base bias, we can control the hole current

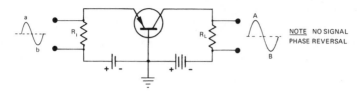

1. ON THE FIRST HALF CYCLE OF THE INPUT (a) THE POSITIVE SIGNAL AIDS FORWARD BIAS INCREASING CURRENT THROUGH THE SYSTEM, CAUSING THE VOLTAGE ACROSS R$_L$ TO INCREASE (A)

2. ON THE SECOND HALF CYCLE OF THE INPUT (b) THE NEGATIVE SIGNAL OPPOSES FORWARD BIAS, DECREASING CIRCUIT CURRENT, CAUSING THE VOLTAGE ACROSS R$_L$ TO DECREASE (B)

Fig. 13-7: Operation of a PNP common base amplifier

through the *PNP* transistor, and consequently electron current in the external circuit.

1. As the input signal swings to its most positive value, this voltage adds to the forward bias at the emitter, resulting in increased hole current through the transistor.

2. This in turn increases external circuit current and the voltage across R_L increases due to the increase in current through R_L *(E = I × R).*

3. As the input signal swings negative, its voltage opposes forward bias, thereby decreasing emitter current.

4. This in turn results in a decrease in collector circuit current and the voltage across R_L therefore decreases.

NOTE: (1) No phase reversal occurs between the input and output signals, a characteristic of all common base amplifiers. Other important facts about C-B amplifiers are: (2) low input impedance, (3) high output impedance, (4) current gain less than 1, and (5) high voltage gain.

The values used to determine the characteristics of impedance are taken with respect to the impedance between the points at which the input and output signals are detected. Since an emitter base junction is forward biased, it reflects a low impedance while the reverse biased base collector junction reflects a high impedance. (For a review of circuit impedance see Chapter 2).

An *NPN* common base amplifier functions in much the same way as a *PNP* with only the current direction and the bias batteries

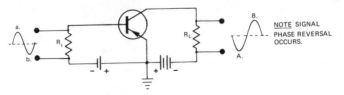

1. ON THE FIRST HALF CYCLE OF THE INPUT (a) THE POSITIVE SIGNAL OPPOSES
   FORWARD BIAS, DECREASING CIRCUIT CURRENT, CAUSING THE VOLTAGE
   ACROSS R_L TO DECREASE (A)
2. ON THE SECOND HALF CYCLE OF THE INPUT (b), THE NEGATIVE SIGNAL AIDS
   FORWARD BIAS, INCREASING CIRCUIT CURRENT, CAUSING THE VOLTAGE
   ACROSS R_L TO INCREASE (B)

Fig. 13-8: Operation of a PNP common emitter amplifier

reversed. This current and bias reversal is true of all three amplifier configurations when a different type transistor is to be considered.

A **common emitter (CE) amplifier** (Figure 13-8) has a much different effect upon the input signal than the common base amplifier. The sequential events that produce amplification are summarized as follows:

E_{in}
(first
half cycle)

1. *E* input swings positive—*opposing forward bias.*
2. Decrease in forward bias = decreased hole current.
3. Decreased transistor hole current = decreased circuit current.
4. Potential across R_L decreases due to decreased current through R_L *(E = I X R).*

E_{in}
(second
half cycle)

5. E_{in} swings negative—aiding forward bias.
6. Increased forward bias = increased hole current.
7. Increased hole current = increased circuit current.
8. Potential across R_L increases due to increased current through R_L *(E = I X R).*

The major difference between this circuit and the one discussed previously is the phase of the output signal. Phase reversal occurs due to injection of the signal at the base (instead of emitter) thereby causing the input voltage to have an opposite effect on forward bias and consequently circuit current.

Additional effects in the CE amplifier are: (1) moderate input impedance; (2) high output impedance; (3) high voltage gain; (4) high current gain (this is due to the current gain being considered as the ratio of a change in collector current to a change in base current).

In the **common collector (CC) amplifier,** the same basic principles of bias change and resulting current changes apply. In a CC amplifier, however, the signal is usually injected at the base and taken out at the emitter (Figure 13-9). The result is a signal with a voltage gain *less than one* and no phase reversal. What use is an amplifier with no gain? Common collector amplifiers are used as impedance matching circuits to match a high impedance circuit to a low impedance circuit. Gain is not a factor in such applications. Since the signal is injected between base and collector (collector is grounded) the reflected input impedance is high while the output circuit, taken emitter to collector, reflects a moderate to low impedance. Another name for a CC amplifier is an *emitter follower.*

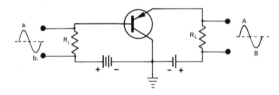

NOTE INPUT IS FED TO THE BASE, OUTPUT TAKEN FROM THE
EMITTER. SINCE THE POTENTIAL ACROSS R$_L$ CANNOT
AT ANY TIME EXCEED THE VALUE OF THE EMITTER–
COLLECTOR BATTERY THE OUTPUT IS NOT AMPLIFIED.

Fig. 13-9: A PNP common collector amplifier

SUMMARY OF IMPORTANT CONCEPTS

If we understand the concepts of bias relating to *PNP* and *NPN* transistors, a ready understanding of transistor amplifier circuits can be developed by following these steps in circuit analysis:

1. Find out what the circuit is supposed to do; *i.e.,* amplify oscillate, etc.
2. Determine the transistor type (*NPN-PNP*).
3. Determine the amplifier class (CB or CE or CC).
4. Determine what the given input signal is doing to forward bias (increasing it or decreasing it).

5. Remember that *increased forward bias* means *increased circuit current* and vice-versa.
6. With reference to step 2, determine what effect the resulting current change will have on the potential at the output point.

By following these steps and taking a little time to analyze transistor circuits, a practical working knowledge of almost any type of circuit may be obtained.

electronic circuits I

CHAPTER 14

In Chapter 11, when we began to discuss special purpose tubes, *interelectrode capacitance* and *feedback* were identified as two factors contributing to the distortion in amplifier output signals under certain conditions. To understand the operation of many of the following circuits, a basic knowledge of the effects of interelectrode capacitance and feedback is necessary.

At high frequencies the interelectrode capacitance found in an amplifier circuit passes a portion of the output signal back into the input circuit. This feedback signal can be either: (a) *regenerative* (in phase with the input, thereby adding to it), or (b) *degenerative* (out of phase with the input and therefore subtracting from it). Regenerative and degenerative feedback are sometimes called, respectively, *positive* and *negative* feedback. In a normal amplifier excessive *re*generative feedback gives a greatly increased gain, but above a certain level, it also causes parasitic "oscillations" to occur and the result is a distorted and unstable output. In contrast, the correct amount of *de*generative feedback can produce a very stable amplifier, but the stability is obtained at the expense of a decrease in gain.

Both forms of feedback are used in different types of electronic circuits, and the first class of circuits we will discuss are called **oscillators**. Oscillator circuits use regenerative feedback to enable them to deliver constant frequency outputs without the use of external input signals. An oscillator is really nothing more than an amplifier that gets its input signal from its own output. Before considering oscillator circuits in detail, we should first look at how electrical oscillations are produced.

OSCILLATIONS AND TANK CIRCUITS

In the study of physics a classical example of an oscillating device is the pendulum. Since the word *oscillator* comes from the latin *oscillare*, meaning *to swing*, the pendulum is an appropriate example. In electronics, a more encompassing definition of oscillation is alternate movement or fluctuations in a system, opposite in direction, around some mean value. From the viewpoint of electrical circuits the application of this definition to alternating current is also very appropriate. The definition implies that any device which produces an AC current is actually an oscillator. This is true; but to simplify matters a little, generators employing electromechanical production of an alternating current are not classed as oscillators. The term *oscillator* is generally reserved for those circuits that transform power from a DC source to produce an oscillating output.

In today's electronic circuitry the oscillator represents one of the most important applications of vacuum tubes and transistors. Oscillator circuits can produce AC signals with constant frequency (and amplitude) ranging from a few cycles per second to several hundred million cycles per second. These circuits find application in innumerable biomedical devices, from audio generators used for testing hearing to ultrasonic generators used in the diagnosis of mitral stenosis or the diathermy equipment used in physical therapy. One basic circuit around which complex oscillators are designed is the **tank circuit.** Two familiar devices, the coil and capacitor, can be used to produce electrical oscillations in a tank circuit (Figure 14-1) as follows:

A. When the switch (A) is placed in position (1) the capacitor charges rapidly to the battery voltage.

With the capacitor fully charged, if the switch is moved to an open position (between (1) and (2), the capacitor will hold the charge.

B. Moving the switch to position (2) gives the capacitor a path for discharge. During discharge a magnetic field builds up around L (14-$1B$). When the capacitor has almost fully discharged, (14-$1C$) the magnetic field will collapse (remember that an inductor opposes a change in current flow).

C. The collapsing field induces current in such a manner as to

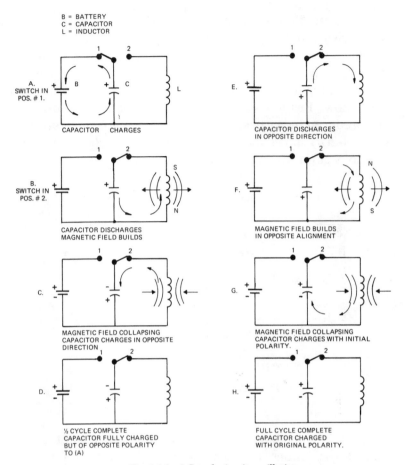

B = BATTERY
C = CAPACITOR
L = INDUCTOR

A.
SWITCH IN
POS. # 1.

CAPACITOR   CHARGES

E.

CAPACITOR DISCHARGES
IN OPPOSITE DIRECTION

B.
SWITCH IN
POS. # 2.

CAPACITOR DISCHARGES
MAGNETIC FIELD BUILDS

F.

MAGNETIC FIELD BUILDS
IN OPPOSITE ALIGNMENT

C.

MAGNETIC FIELD COLLAPSING
CAPACITOR CHARGES IN OPPOSITE
DIRECTION

G.

MAGNETIC FIELD COLLAPSING
CAPACITOR CHARGES WITH INITIAL
POLARITY.

D.

½ CYCLE COMPLETE
CAPACITOR FULLY CHARGED
BUT OF OPPOSITE POLARITY
TO (A)

H.

FULL CYCLE COMPLETE
CAPACITOR CHARGED
WITH ORIGINAL POLARITY.

Fig. 14-1: LC tank circuit oscillations   •

oppose the decrease in capacitor discharging current, thereby acting as a generator and charging the capacitor in the opposite direction (14-1*D*).

D. When the magnetic field has collapsed completely, there is nothing holding the charge on the capacitor and it can therefore discharge. Its discharge path is again through *L* (14-1*E*), but in the *opposite* direction, thereby building up an oppositely polarized magnetic field (14-1*F*).

E. With the capacitor again almost fully discharged, the magnetic field once more collapses (14-1*G*), inducing a current flow such that the capacitor will charge with its original polarity (14-1*H*).

If there were no resistance in the circuit to cause losses of energy, this circuit would be a perpetual motion device. However, losses do occur and the result is an eventual damping of the circuit current flow. Figure 14-2 (*A*) shows the relative portions of the signal produced by a capacitor and coil in an *ideal* (no loss) circuit. Figure 14-2(*B*) shows the output from a *practical* circuit in which losses do occur, resulting in a damped signal.

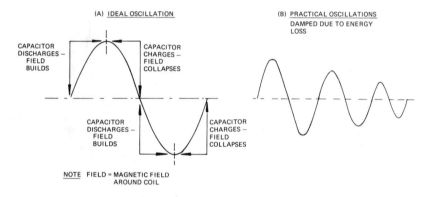

Fig. 14-2: Ideal versus practical oscillations

From this discussion it is obvious that we cannot produce sustained oscillations by charging the tank circuit only once. Energy lost on each cycle must be replaced in order to maintain a constant amplitude signal. This could be done in Figure 14-1, step (*H*), by, at that time, throwing the switch to position (*1*), thereby allowing the capacitor to draw the needed energy from the battery. This periodic addition of "regenerating" energy is commonly known as **regenerative feedback**. Since employing a mechanical switch at high frequencies is limiting and impractical, another method of obtaining this regenerative energy must be available. We can solve this problem by using a vacuum tube (or transistor) amplifier as a switch (alternately driving it below cut-off and back) and a transformer to give phase reversal. The tickler coil oscillator is an example of this type of circuit.

Tickler Coil Oscillator

Remembering that a signal phase shift of 180° occurs from grid to plate in a vacuum tube, and also across a transformer (primary to secondary) we can analyze the **tickler coil oscillator circuit** (Figure 14-3).

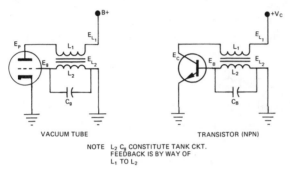

VACUUM TUBE   TRANSISTOR (NPN)

NOTE L_2 C_g CONSTITUTE TANK CKT.
FEEDBACK IS BY WAY OF
L_1 TO L_2

Fig. 14-3: Tickler coil oscillators

L_2 and C_g form the grid tank circuit of the oscillator. Any voltage change (E_g) in the grid tank circuit is felt at the plate 180° out of phase (E_P). The same change will be reflected in L_1 (E_{L_1}) since it is in series with the tube. Any fluctuations produced in L_1 will be shifted 180° when induced into L_2 (E_{L_2}) and therefore return to the grid *in phase* with the original signal. This regenerative plate feedback sustains the oscillations in the tank circuit so that they will be constant in amplitude. The summarized voltage changes can be shown as follows:

(1) E_g ⎱
                 ⎰ 180° phase shift
(2) E_P ⎱
                 ⎰ in phase
(3) E_{L_1} ⎱
                 ⎰ 180° phase shift
(4) E_{L_2} ⎰

The two shifts of 180° each have the total effect that E_{L_2} is in phase with E_g.

We can now summarize the requirements for a sustained output oscillator:

1. A DC power source.

2. A switching device (vacuum tube of transistor).

3. A frequency determining device (tank circuit or RC circuit).

4. Regenerative feedback.

The tickler coil oscillator just discussed could also have been called a *tuned grid oscillator* since the frequency determining device (resonant tank) was in the grid circuit. The frequency determining device could just as well have been placed in the plate circuit, in which case the oscillator would be referred to as a *tuned plate oscillator*.

Crystal Controlled Oscillators

Certain natural crystals under conditions of mechanical stress produce an electrical charge difference across their structure. Conversely, when an electrical charge is placed across such a crystal, it is mechanically distorted. This phenomenon is known as the **piezoelectric effect** (*c.f.* Chapter 17). The distortion of a dielectric was mentioned previously in the study of capacitors. The same principle effect is cumulative within a crystal and thereby distorts the whole structure. Every crystal has its own frequency of natural, mechanical resonance. If an applied voltage is of the same frequency, the natural distortions are reinforced by those of the electric field, and the mechanical vibrations and crystal current are maximum. Under these conditions a crystal mounted between two plates as shown in Figure 14-4 (*A*) has an equivalent electrical circuit to that shown in Figure 14-4 (*B*). C_1 represents the electrode capacitance, while L, C_2, and R represent the electrical vibrating material. A crystal is able to function as the electrical equivalent of an LC tank circuit and thus may be used in many

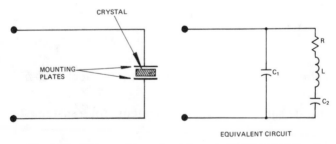

Fig. 14-4: A mounted crystal and its equivalent electrical circuit

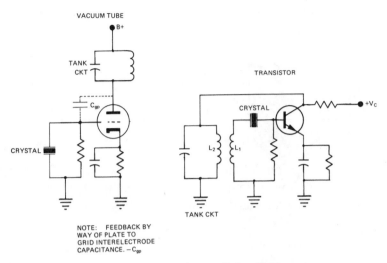

Fig. 14-5: Crystal controlled oscillators

oscillator circuits as well as filter networks. Crystals make exceptionally good oscillator circuits since they have very low energy dissipation and minimal dependence on other circuit characteristics such as amplification factor, plate resistance, aging of tubes, and DC supply fluctuations, making the circuit's output extremely stable. Figure 14-5 shows schematic diagrams for typical crystal-controlled oscillators. Feedback in the vacuum tube oscillator is produced by tube interelectrode capacitances shown by (C_{gp}).

A Hartley Oscillator

If instead of individual primary and secondary coils, a center tapped coil is used as an auto-transformer, a tickler coil oscillator becomes a **Hartley oscillator**. Hartley oscillators operate at high radio frequencies (RF) while tickler coil oscillators are more adequate generally at low (audio) frequencies. Figure 14-6 shows typical Hartley oscillators. The vacuum tube circuit operates as follows: L-L_1 and C function as the tank circuit, and the feedback is fed from L to L_1 to maintain oscillations. Since the DC current path of the tube runs through a portion of the tank circuit (L), the oscillator is called a *series-fed* Hartley. An RF choke is used to

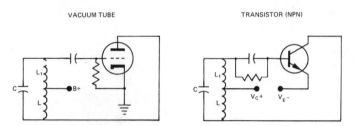

Fig. 14-6: Hartley oscillators (series fed)

block RF energy out of the power supply. When the DC current path does not flow through *any* portion of the tank circuit, the oscillator is *shunt-fed* Hartley (Figure 14-7).

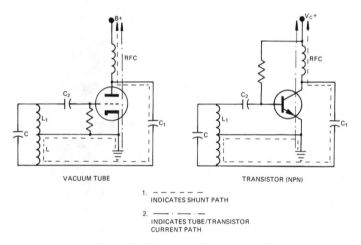

1. – – – – – –
INDICATES SHUNT PATH

2. — · — · —
INDICATES TUBE/TRANSISTOR
CURRENT PATH

Fig. 14-7: Hartley oscillators - shunt fed.

Phase Shift Oscillators

Inductive-capacitive tank circuits are not the only method of producing oscillation, as was seen in the discussion of the crystal oscillator. A third type of practical oscillator, and one that is widely employed, is the *RC* (resistive-capacitive) coupled oscillator. From the study of capacitors we learned that a lag in voltage, relative to its circuit current, occurs across a capacitor (ICE). If we place a resistor in the charge current path (and since current and voltage relative to a resistor are in phase), a resistive voltage drop *leading* that across the capacitor can be obtained. By selecting the use of three *RC* networks, each causing a voltage phase shift of 60°, a total phase shift of 180° can be produced across the whole network. Figure 14-8 shows an *RC* phase-shift oscillator. Below each *RC* network is a vector representative of the phase angle of the voltage. If we drive the tube or transistor in the circuit alternately to saturation and then cut off, oscillations are sustained, and a constant-frequency constant-amplitude output signal is obtained.

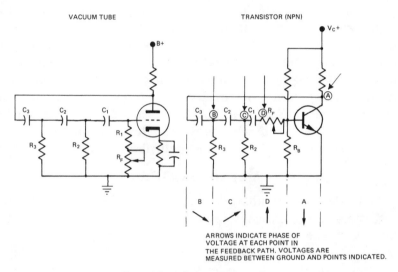

Fig. 14-8: RC phase shift oscillators

SUMMARY OF IMPORTANT CONCEPTS

The four basic requirements for any oscillator circuit are (1) *DC power source,* (2) a *switching device,* (3) a *frequency determining device,* and (4) *regenerative feedback.* Common frequency determining devices are *L-C "tanks," R-C circuits,* and *crystals.* Regenerative feedback is accomplished by (a) *transformer action* (Tickler and Hartley oscillators), (b), *RC phase shifting* (phase shift oscillators) or (c) *inter-electrode capacitances* (crystal oscillators). By varying the value of any component in the *frequency determining network,* the frequency of oscillation can be changed.

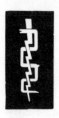

electronic circuits II

CHAPTER 15

CLASSIFICATION OF OSCILLATORS

The most convenient method for classifying oscillators is based on an examination of their output waveforms. Circuits having sinusoidal outputs are classed as **sinusoidal oscillators**, while the many circuits that produce outputs other than sinusoidal can be placed under the loose classification of **non-sinusoidal oscillators**. An important group of circuits characterized by outputs that change *suddenly* from one state to another (*i.e.,* from saturation to cut-off) are called **relaxation oscillators**. The most common type of relaxation oscillator is the **multivibrator**.

MULTIVIBRATORS

Multivibrators are subdivided into three groups: (1) free running (or **astable**); (2) one-shot (or **monostable**); and (3) flip-flop (or **bistable**). These circuits consist of two amplifiers, coupled together in such a way that the output of one is used as the input of the second, and vice-versa. They operate by alternately switching each other on or off, and the output signal is obtained from the plate (or collector in the case of transistor circuits) of one of the amplifiers. By the selection of the correct circuit components used to couple the two amplifiers, many types of output waveforms can be developed. These outputs can vary from discrete individual pulses to continuous symmetrical square waves. Figure 15-1 shows three possible multivibrator output waveforms.

The **free running** or **astable multivibrator** is characterized by continual switching of its two amplifiers, alternately *on* and *off* (when one is *on,* the other is *off*). The output is a symmetrical *square wave* or rectangular wave (Figure 15-1*A*).

The **one shot** or **monostable multivibrator** remains in one predetermined stable state (one amplifier *on,* the other *off*) until

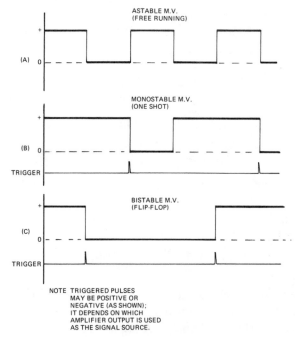

Fig. 15-1: Multivibrator waveforms

triggered, at which time it switches to the opposite condition for a designated time, and then returns to its original stable state again. The output is a *pulse* of predetermined duration (Figure 15-1*B*).

The **flip-flop** or **bistable multivibrator** is stable in either condition until triggered (either one of the amplifiers can be *on*). When a trigger signal is applied, the two amplifiers switch their *off-on* states and remain that way until triggered again to return to their original conditions. The output voltage switches back and forth (when triggered) between two possible steady state DC values (Figure 15-1*C*).

Astable Multivibrator Action

Whether tube-type or transistorized, the basic operation of multivibrators is the same. By examination of a typical circuit, the basic principles of the multivibrator action can be summarized. In Figure 15-2, Figure (*A*) is a block diagram of a **free running (astable) plate-coupled multivibrator**; Figure (*B*) is the schematic.

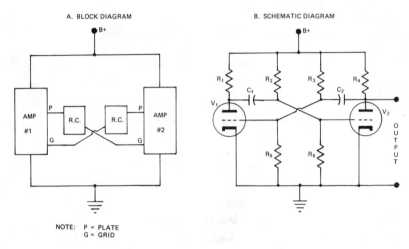

NOTE: P = PLATE
        G = GRID

Fig. 15-2: An astable (free running) multivibrator

The plate (output) signals are fed back, through *RC* networks, to the opposite amplifier inputs. A most important fact to be remembered is that *grid and plate signals* in an amplifier (base and collector signals in the case of a *CE* transistor circuit) are *180° out of phase.*

A typical switching sequence occurs as follows:

1. When V_1 swings toward saturation, its output goes in a negative direction.
2. This change coupled through the *RC* network is felt at V_2 input.
3. A negative swing at the input tends to drive V_2 to cut-off. Therefore, its output (plate) swings positive.
4. This positive swing coupled back to V_1 input drives it fully to saturation.

Each amplifier will now remain in this condition for a set amount of time due to the action of the capacitors in the *RC* networks. V_2 is held at cut-off by a discharging capacitor reflecting a *negative* voltage at its input; with V_1 the effects of the capacitor and potential are reversed, causing V_1 to stay in saturation. As soon as the capacitors cease their charging or discharging activity, a switch to the opposite state occurs. The switching action is as follows:

1. When the capacitor holding V_2 cut-off is fully discharged, the

negative input at V_2 is removed and the grid goes positive (zero relative to a negative value represents a positive change).

2. This positive going input causes V_2 to swing into conduction and its output (plate) voltage begins to swing negative.

3. The negative swing coupled back to V_1 input causes it to move from saturation toward cut-off.

4. V_1 output (plate) therefore swings positive and, coupled back to V_2 input, drives V_2 into saturation.

The amplifiers remain in this state (the reverse of their previous condition) until the capacitors stop their activity and the whole sequence starts over again. The output, taken from one or the other of the amplifiers, is a rectangular wave, alternately changing from a high DC voltage to a low DC voltage and back again, as shown in Figure 15-3. Changing the value of resistance or capacitance in the RC coupling networks varies conduction or cut-off times, resulting in waveforms like those shown in Figure 15-4.

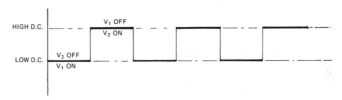

Fig. 15-3: Output waveform from an astable multivibrator - taken off V_1 plate

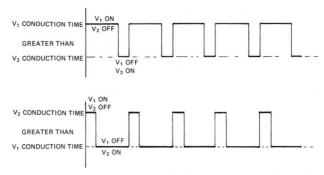

Fig. 15-4: Results of varying conduction times of a free running multivibrator by changing the values of R and C in the coupling circuits.

Monostable Multivibrators

Monostable multivibrators have one stable condition in which they remain fixed until triggered. Figure 15-5A shows a monostable circuit. The normal condition of the circuit is V_1 cut-off, V_2 conducting. Application of a positive trigger at V_1 grid starts it conducting, causing its plate voltage to swing negative. C_F (previously charged to the potential at V_1 plate) must therefore discharge through R_F, placing a negative at V_2 grid. This cuts off V_2 during C_F discharge. V_2 plate voltage is at a high potential during this time, keeping V_1 conducting. When C_F has fully discharged, the negative potential is removed from V_2 grid, it can now conduct, and its plate voltage swings negative. The negative swing, coupled to V_1 grid, drives V_1 once again to cut-off, and the stable condition is reached. Notice that the circuit only gives an output pulse when triggered.

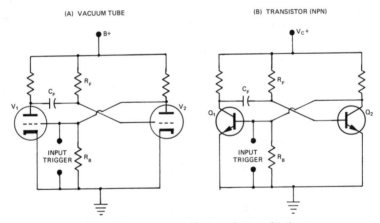

Fig. 15-5: A monostable (one-shot) multivibrator

The action described is virtually the same whether the circuit is a vacuum tube or transistor. Replacing the two tubes in Figure 15-5A with two NPN grounded emitter transistors (Figure 15-5B) will yield a similar operation.

Bistable Multivibrators

Bistable multivibrators (or, as they are sometimes called, flip-flop circuits) are used extensively in computers and therefore

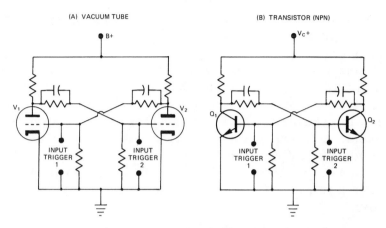

Fig. 15-6: A bistable (flip-flop) multivibrator

deserve mention. A bistable multivibrator as shown in Figure 15-6*A* is stable in either of two states; V_1 conducting, V_2 cut-off—or V_1 cut-off, V_2 conducting. In Figure 15-6 we will consider V_1 to be *on* (conducting) and V_2 to be off (cut-off). A negative going trigger at the input will cause V_1 to decrease conduction, with a resulting positive swing of its plate potential. This positive going signal, coupled to V_2 grid, causes it to begin conducting. Its plate voltage therefore swings negative; V_1 grid follows, driving V_1 to cut-off.

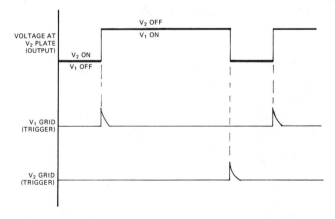

Fig. 15-7: Input triggers and output waveform of a bistable (flip-flop) multivibrator.

The system will remain this way until a positive going trigger at
V_1 grid (or a negative at V_2 grid) initiates the reverse sequence,
and the circuit returns to its original condition.

Figure 15-7 shows the output waveform of a typical flip-flop
multivibrator. Just as with the monostable circuit, the bistable
circuit tubes could be replaced by *NPN* grounded emitter
transistors (Figure 15-6B) with little change in the basic operating
concept. Although similar in construction to the astable multivibrator, the difference between the flip-flop and the bistable
multivibrator is that the conduction/cut-off time in the bistable
circuit is dependent, *not* on *RC* networks, but on the input
triggers.

A RAMP FUNCTION (SAWTOOTH) GENERATOR

The circuits in this and the next section are not oscillators in
the strict sense of the word, but the waveforms they generate are
widely used, which makes them too important to be omitted.

A voltage that increases at a linear rate with respect to time is
called a **ramp function voltage**. A circuit which produces such a
waveform repeatedly is consequently termed a **ramp function
generator**. These circuits are used in all types of oscilloscopes to
drive the electron beam back and forth across its screen as well as
in many other special applications.

Many different designs of ramp function generators are possible,
from vacuum tube and transistor types to thyratrons (see
appendix for definition) and neon tube circuits. Figure 15-8 shows

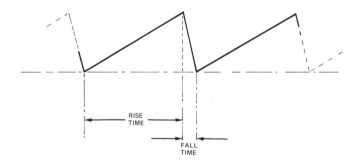

Fig. 15-8: A ramp voltage waveform

one cycle of a typical (sawtooth) ramp function waveform. The two time periods are designated **rise time** (voltage increasing) and **fall time** (voltage decreasing). Notice that the fall time is *much* shorter than the rise time. (The electron beam on an oscilloscope moves relatively slowly left to right across the screen, but very rapidly right to left. If the relationship between this action and the sawtooth waveform is not clear, review Chapter 11 for a detailed explanation.)

Most ramp function generators use a capacitor to develop the output voltage of the circuit. Since capacitors charge at an exponential rate (Chapter 7), in order to obtain a relatively linear charge rate only a small portion (1/100 of its overall charge curve is used. Figure 15-9 (*A*) shows a capacitor charge curve. The small portion shown between arrows is utilized in obtaining the ramp voltage. By automatically discharging the capacitor each time it reaches the potential of point (*A*), the process is continually repeated and a sawtooth wave results. This is shown in Figure 15-9(*B*).

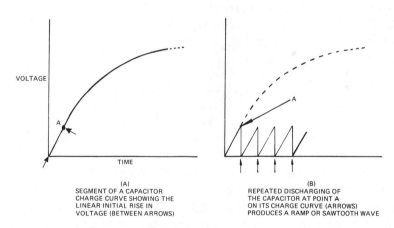

(A)
SEGMENT OF A CAPACITOR
CHARGE CURVE SHOWING THE
LINEAR INITIAL RISE IN
VOLTAGE (BETWEEN ARROWS)

(B)
REPEATED DISCHARGING OF
THE CAPACITOR AT POINT A
ON ITS CHARGE CURVE (ARROWS)
PRODUCES A RAMP OR SAWTOOTH WAVE

Fig. 15-9: Ramp (or sawtooth) waveform generation by selectively triggering a capacitor on the linear part of its charge curve

A typical transistorized ramp function generator is shown in Figure 15-10. The circuit operates as follows:

1. When no input trigger (positive going) is present, the transitor is cut off and the voltage at (*A*) is high.

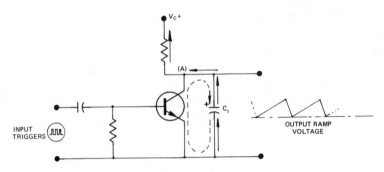

Fig. 15-10: A ramp function (sawtooth) generator

2. C_1 attempts to charge as shown by the solid line to the potential at (A).
3. A positive trigger at the input turns the transistor on (Why?*), giving C_1 a path for discharge as shown by the dotted line.
4. As soon as the trigger is removed from the input, the transistor turns off again (Why?**), and C_1 again begins to charge. The process is repeated.

In Figure 15-9, notice that unless an input trigger occurs at the right moment, the charge rate and the resulting voltage developed could become nonlinear.

A SCHMITT TRIGGER

In modern day electronics and instrumentation, one is often confronted with terms such as *digital readout, digital counter* or *analog to digital converter.* The word *digital* refers to pulse type waveforms (primarily rectangular) used to represent discrete units of information. Since much information obtained in medical applications of electronics is analog in nature, (curves, peaks, *etc.*), and since the trend in newer instruments is toward digital read-out systems we must have a way to convert this information into digital form. One circuit that can be applied in a number of different ways is the **Schmitt trigger**. Application of a sine wave

---

*Application of the positive trigger satisfies the conditions for forward bias across the emitter-base, causing conduction.
**Removal of the trigger removes the forward bias, cutting off the transistor.

signal into a Schmitt trigger results in a square wave output of identical frequency. Figure 15-11(*A*) shows both the input and output signals for such application. Figure 15-11(*B*) shows input and output waveforms for application of a Schmitt trigger as a threshold detector (as found in the Coulter electronic particle counter).

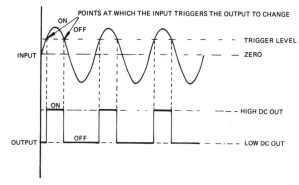

Fig. 15-11(A): Waveforms in a Schmitt trigger circuit changing a sine wave to a rectangular wave of the same frequency

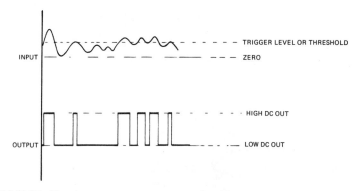

Fig. 15-11(B): Waveforms in a Schmitt trigger circuit functioning as a threshold detector

The operation of a Schmitt trigger circuit is based on the following points:

1. The circuit is capable of two output levels, high and low.
2. With the input signal below a present voltage (the trigger point), the low output is generated.

3. As soon as the input reaches or goes beyond the preset potential, the output immediately swings to its high value.

4. The output remains at this value until the input voltage drops below the preset trigger point, at which time the output returns to its low value.

The result is shown in detail in Figure 15-12(A), while a circuit for producing such a wave form is shown in Figure 15-12(B). In the stable (no-input) condition, Q_1 is cut off, due to the positive potential at the emitter (generated across resistor R_B), reverse biasing the junction, and Q_2 conducting due to forward bias is developed across R_E. A positive (trigger) input at Q_1 base *must exceed* the Q_1 emitter potential in order for the transistor to

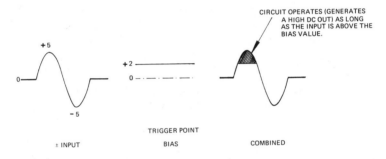

Fig. 15-12(A):   Schmitt trigger bias

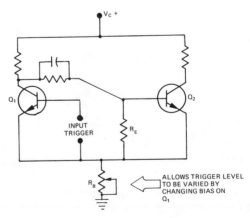

Fig. 15-12(B): A Schmitt trigger circuit with adjustable triggering capability

conduct. As soon as this occurs, the resulting negative swing in the potential at Q_1 collector, coupled to Q_2 base, causes Q_2 to cut off. The collector of Q_2 will then reflect a high potential until the input potential at Q_1 *base* drops below the *emitter* voltage, thereby cutting Q_1 off. At this time the resulting positive swing at Q_1 collector again turns Q_2 on, causing its collector potential to drop once more to its lower ambient value.

The trigger point of Q_1 can be varied by adjusting resistor R_B. This in turn changes the emitter potential that must be overcome by the input signal in order to trigger the system. The circuit is then a *threshold detector*, capable of accepting inputs above a certain level and rejecting all others.

SUMMARY OF CIRCUITS

Oscillators can be classified as **sinusoidal** or **non-sinusoidal** (including relaxation oscillators) based on the type of output signal produced.

Multivibrators are an important form of rectangular wave generating relaxation oscillators. They fall into three general groups:

1. **Free running (astable)** producing a continuous rectangular wave output.
2. **One-shot (monostable)** producing a single rectangular pulse when triggered.
3. **Flip-flop (bistable)** producing either of two stable DC states.

Ramp function generators are characterized by production of a sawtooth-shaped waveform developed by alternately charging and discharging a capacitor within the linear segment of its charge curve.

A **Schmitt trigger** is capable of transforming a sinusoidal or analog input into a digital, square wave, or rectangular wave output.

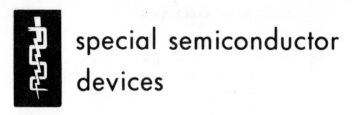

special semiconductor devices

CHAPTER 16

FIELD EFFECT TRANSISTORS

In Chapter 2, the effects of circuit loading on signal sources and power supplies were discussed. It was shown that in order *not* to load a signal source, the circuit acting as the load must reflect a high impedance. Since generally all small signal voltages must first be amplified before they are of a useful magnitude, the load on a signal source is usually an amplifier, and an amplifier used in this way must have a *high input impedance.*

Prior to the advent of transistors, vacuum tube electrometers (see glossary) were used for this purpose. However, today these vacuum tube circuits are being replaced by a relatively new device with an extremely high input impedance: the **field effect transistor (FET).** Used in many modern instruments as an input amplifier or pre-amplifier, a semiconductor FET functions by employing only one type of charge carrier, and by using an electrostatic field to

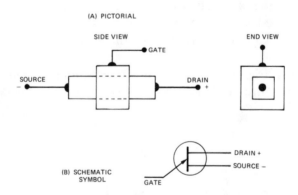

Fig. 16-1: A field effect transistor (FET). (Courtesy Philco-Ford Corp., Tech. Rep. Division, Fort Washington, Pennsylvania)

154

control the flow of these carriers. Figure 16-1 shows two pictorial views of a FET as well as its schematic symbol. The sleeve around the N-type channel crystal serves the same function as the grid in a vacuum tube, and is called the **gate**. Current through the device is produced by way of electron carriers migrating from source (-) to drain (+). By application of a negative potential to the sleeve (or gate), the area beneath the sleeve in the N-type crystal can be made deficient in charge carriers, producing what is known as a **depletion zone**. The fewer the charge carriers in the depletion zone, the less the current flow from source to drain. Consequently, by varying the negative gate potential, source-to-drain current can also be controlled. (The action is similar to that produced by a vacuum tube's control grid.) If a load resistor is placed in series with the FET and a signal applied to the gate (as in Figure 16-2), the current through the system will vary, causing fluctuations in the voltage across the load resistor and reproduction of the signal. This device operates very similarly to a conventional vacuum tube in amplifying a signal, with the exception that the gate draws virtually no current from the signal source, thereby reflecting a very high impedance. This is in contrast to conventional amplifiers which do draw some current from the signal source.

The advantages of a FET are very high input impedance (as high as 10^{10} ohms for MOSFETs) and excellent frequency response (up to 110 MHz or 150 MHz); their principal disadvantages are noise and temperature-induced drift.

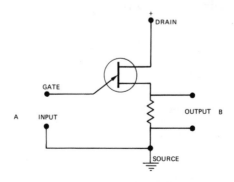

Fig. 16-2: A simple FET circuit

SILICON CONTROLLED RECTIFIERS

A device commonly used as a switch in controlling large amounts of current flow is the **silicon-controlled rectifier** (SCR), which is basically a double junction diode. Figure 16-3 shows pictorial and schematic representatives of a SCR. Note that it is a *PNPN* junction transistor. The second *P* section has a dual role since it acts as a gate and also as one half of the diode formed by the middle *N* and *P* sections (called the *middle diode*). The SCR functions as follows:

1. With voltage applied across the SCR so that the anode is (+) and the cathode (-), and with no input present at the gate, the rectifier will not conduct since the *middle* diode is *reverse biased.*

2. Application of a positive pulse (exceeding the anode potential) to the gate will "turn on" the middle diode, resulting in conduction through the rectifier.

3. Once there is conduction, since the gate no longer has any control, the SCR acts like a conventional diode. This condition is maintained until the cathode/anode current is interrupted or drops below a set value called the **holding current**. When such a current drop occurs, the rectifier shuts off.

4. Once shut off occurs, another input pulse to the gate is required to initiate the sequence again.

Silicon-controlled rectifiers are widely used in power supplies (and psychedelic lighting systems) as controlled current sources, their major advantage being that they enable small current values (gate currents) to control high currents (rectifier currents).

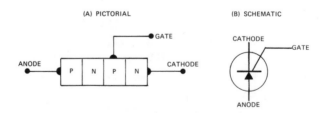

Fig. 16-3:   A silicon-controlled rectifier (SCR). (Courtesy Philco-Ford Corp., Tech. Rep. Division, Fort Washington, Pennsylvania)

ZENER DIODES

Conventional junction diodes, when forward biased, will conduct, but they will not conduct with reverse bias (except for a small amount of minority carrier current). If, however, the diode's reverse breakdown voltage level is exceeded, a sudden surge of avalanche current flows, the junction is destroyed, and the diode ruined. Because of this, circuit designers are careful to insure that a junction diode operates well below its characteristic breakdown potential.

A unique type of semiconductor diode, which actually uses avalanche current for normal operation, is the **Zener diode.** Whereas avalanche current will normally ruin a conventional junction diode, it does not affect a Zener diode as long as the current value is kept within certain limits. This unique property of Zener diodes is due to a characteristic designed into them, called **silicon resistivity** (excess impurities). Correct manufacturing can produce a Zener diode which will operate at almost any desired breakdown voltage (the breakdown voltage in Zener diodes is generally called the *Zener voltage.*)

Zener diodes are used extensively as voltage regulators and reference voltage sources. Operated at the Zener point, there is constant voltage across the diode, while the current through it can be varied over a relatively wide range.

Figure 16-4 shows the schematic symbol for a Zener diode and its voltage/current curve. Note that at the Zener point a fixed

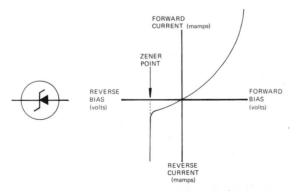

Fig. 16-4: A Zener diode schematic symbol and characteristic curve

voltage can be obtained even though the current may vary in magnitude.

TUNNEL DIODES

Ordinary junction diodes operate mainly with forward bias, while Zener diodes operate under reverse bias. A third type of *PN* junction diode is available which operates in its own unique way, at times (depending upon circuit design) as an amplifier or at other times as an oscillator: this is the **tunnel diode**. The usual current flow across a *PN* junction results from the effects of forward and reverse bias, and is referred to as *diffusion current*. A phenomenon known as *tunneling* results from the special design of a tunnel diode. Another form of current (*tunnel current*) occurs in these devices and it is explained by the principles of quantum mechanics. This tunnel current, in conjunction with normal diffusion current, produces the unique operating characteristics of the tunnel diode. Figure 16-5 shows typical voltage/current curves for a normal diode and a tunnel diode. On one part of the curve for the tunnel diode, forward current *decreases* as forward bias *increases*. This area is known as the *negative resistance region*. By operating the diode in this region, it can be made to function as an amplifier or even as an oscillator.

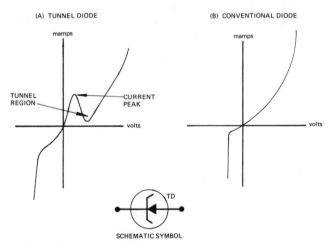

Fig. 16-5: Voltage/current characteristic curves of a tunnel diode and a conventional diode

Tunnel diodes are capable of operating at frequencies in excess of 500 MHz and are useful as switching devices in computer circuitry.

INTEGRATED CIRCUITS

Integrated circuits are the newest elements finding application in today's instruments. These microelectronic devices, as small or in some cases many times smaller than some transistors, yet are complete circuits containing both active elements (transistors) and passive elements (capacitors, resistors). These extremely compact circuits can be classified into three different groups, based on their method of construction: **solid-state** (or **monolithic**) **circuits, thin-film circuits**, and **high density circuits**.

Although any transistorized circuit can be referred to in a general way as a "solid state" circuit, it is better to reserve the name *solid-state* for the **monolithic circuits**, which are manufactured from a single crystal of silicon *P* or *N* type material that is first photo-etched and then doped a number of times with the appropriate "road map" of circuit elements. By inclusion of several stages of amplification within one package, various complex circuits such as DC amplifiers, oscillators, multivibrators, *etc.*, can be constructed from a single crystal element with appropriate external components.

Of the two other types of integrated circuits, **thin-layer circuits** are the next closest to being solid-state. These circuits are constructed by depositing various materials upon a glass substrate, in layers. The conductive and active elements are then separated from each other by nonconductive coatings, and the circuit is placed in a transistor case or some similar container. Just as with monolithic circuits, thin-layer packages can have multiple applications, determined by the external components used with them.

High density circuits are constructed from individual microcomponents that are connected together and placed in a conventional transistor shell or container.

The trend today is in the direction of even smaller, more compact, and efficient monolithic circuits. An example of the biomedical use of these devices is the *endo-radiosonde,* a pill containing a microtransmitter than can be surgically implanted or even swallowed to transmit diagnostic information. Only the future will tell what future advances in microelectronics will bring.

The advantages of these microcircuits over conventional transistors parallel the advantages of transistors when compared with vacuum tubes: extremely high reliability, small size, and low power requirements.

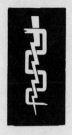

SECTION II

clinical analytical
instrumentation

transducers

CHAPTER 17

ENERGY CLASSES AND BASIC TRANSDUCERS

Any device that is capable of converting one form of energy into another is a **transducer**. There are a multitude of different types and designs of transducers but the parameters they measure can be condensed into five (somewhat arbitrary) classes based on the type of energy involved: **mechanical, thermal, chemical, optical,** and **nuclear.** These five energy classes are by no means strict; many of the measurable parameters overlap. For example, a force producing linear displacement (*movement*) is physically the same form of true energy as a force resulting in mechanical distortion (*pressure*). However, a different type of transducer is required to measure each action. In effect, the classifications are more of a working convenience than a true tabulation of different energy forms.

In this chapter we will examine some highly simplified examples of electrical output transducers commonly found in medical applications (diagnostic, analytical and therapeutic). To cover this material in anything but a superficial way would require a book in itself; therefore, the interested reader is referred to references in the appendix for more detailed information.

Based on the five energy classes, electrical output transducers can be referred to as mechanoelectric, thermoelectric, etc., since they accept an input of energy from one of the five classes and produce an electrical output signal. These devices can take one of two operating forms, based on the number of inputs required. A **self-generating** or **active** transducer is one which requires only a single (or primary) input to produce an output. (One example is a photocell in which a pulse of light in gives an electrical pulse out). A **passive** transducer on the other hand requires two or more inputs: a driving or operating (secondary) input and the detected (or primary) input to produce an output. A typical example of a

163

passive transducer is a vacuum or gas phototube. The secondary input (power supply voltage) makes the tube active while the primary input (changes in light intensity) causes variation in the current flow through the tube.

Theoretically, any type of energy can be utilized for either the input or output of a transducer. This chapter, however, will consider only transducers with outputs that are electrical in nature (variations in resistance, current, or voltage).

MECHANOELECTRIC TRANSDUCERS

Any phenomenon that falls under the laws of motion, gravity, conservation of momentum, or energy can be detected by an appropriate mechanoelectric transducer. A few mechanical parameters for which transducers have been designed are:

1. Displacement—linear or angular;
2. Pressure—absolute, relative or differential;
3. Torque;
4. Velocity;
5. Acceleration—linear or angular;
6. Dimensional variations.

A very simple example of a widely used transducer using a mechanoelectric relationship is the **mercury strain gauge** (Figure 17-1). A change in its dimension acts as the input, producing a change in resistance as an output, (*i.e.,* it is mechanoresistive). In the discussion of resistors we found that the resistance of a conductor is a function of its resistivity, cross-sectional area, and length. By decreasing its cross-sectional area *or* increasing length,

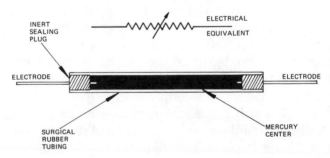

Fig. 17-1: A simple mercury strain gauge and its electrical equivalent circuit

the resistance of a conductor is increased; and vice versa. This characteristic of varying resistance is used in the design of both electrolytic and mercury strain gauges. In the mercury strain gauge a small-diameter rubber tube (surgical rubber) is filled with mercury and sealed at each end by electrodes. As the tube is stretched, the diameter decreases, the length increases, and consequently the resistance is increased. Similar gauges are used to measure pulse rates, respiration rates, and even kidney volume changes. The mercury strain gauge acts as a passive transducer since, to detect the resistance change (primary signal), a current (secondary signal) must first flow through the system.

A second example of a mechanoelectric transducer employs the principle of the **piezo-electric effect** in its operation. Mechanical distortions of certain crystalline materials (quartz SiO_2) or Rochelle salt) set up stresses within the lattice structure that result in polarization of charges on the surface of the crystal (Figure 17-2). This action is reversible since application of a voltage across the same crystal will produce mechanical distortion. The combined reversible effects are referred to as the piezo-electric effect.

Any force capable of distorting a piezo-crystal, (pressure, bending, etc.) will result in production of a voltage that can be measured. This fact is utilized in the application of these crystals as transducers in phonograph pick-ups, microphones, earphones, and even pressure-sensitive pulse detectors.

Since quartz and Rochelle salt are dependent upon correct

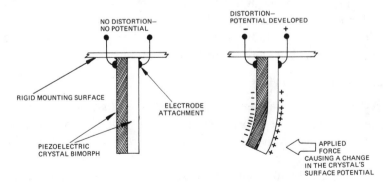

Fig. 17-2: Simplified diagram showing the piezoelectric effect

cutting and orientation to yield satisfactory results, piezo elements manufactured as molded ceramics of **barium titanate** constructed to required specifications are being widely used in their place. The sensitivity of these molded elements is less than that of natural piezo devices, but they are (1) cheaper than quartz, and (2) have a wider stable temperature range than Rochelle salt.

A recent application of piezo-electric transducers in the field of ultrasonic diagnosis and therapy is their use to transmit and/or receive elements in pulsed ultrasonic generators. Ultrasound is used in the detection of such medical problems as pericardial effusion and mitral valve disease, and the location of intracranial tumors. The basic procedure consists of transmitting focused sound into the diseased part of the body and analyzing the echo signals that result. This procedure is further discussed in Chapter 21; the therapeutic use of ultrasound is discussed in Chapter 27.

THERMOELECTRIC TRANSDUCERS

Although thermal, optical, and nuclear transducers can all be grouped under the single heading of radiation transducers, they are best discussed separately under their specialized applications. This section deals with transducers that detect change in temperature, yielding electrical outputs.

Temperature transducers fall into two basic groups: those showing a resistance change (**thermoresistive**) and those producing a voltage (**thermocouples**). Thermoresistive transducers are temperature-sensing elements that can be either (1) metallic or (2) semiconductor in nature. Thermocouples are voltage-generating metallic devices. Other types of temperature-measuring devices can be found that use inductance or capacitance as their electrical output variable, but they are not widely used.

Thermoresistive Devices

As the name implies, thermoresistive transducers exhibit a change in resistance when exposed to a changing temperature. Metallic thermoresistive elements have a *positive temperature coefficient;* their resistance increases with an increase in temperature. On the other hand, semiconductors (and electrolyte solutions) have a *negative temperature coefficient;* their resistance decreases with an increase in temperature. Semiconductor temperature transducers can be one of two types: true thermoresistive devices called *thermistors* (*thermally*-sensitive *resistors*) or heat-sensitive silicon *junction diodes*. (The latter group of transducers could be considered as a separate class entirely, but for simplicity they will be listed as semiconductor thermoresistive elements).

A. Metallic Resistance Transducers

The temperature-resistance relationship of metals is dependent mainly upon their purity since pure materials have high positive temperature coefficients, while alloys exhibit lower (or even negative) coefficients. Although the relationship between resistance and temperature is a linear one over a certain range (characteristic of the metal), at higher temperatures this characteristic is rapidly lost as is illustrated in Figure 17-3 which shows the relative temperature-resistance curves for two wires of nickel and platinum having the same resistance at zero degrees centigrade.

Metallic resistance transducers commonly take one of three forms: (a) wire grids, (b) wire coils, and (c) metal ribbons. The form of the element is usually dictated by the application desired but in practically all instances a support medium of insulating material is used and, in some cases, a protective tube or cover (glass or metal) is required. Since metals are classed as good conductors, high resistive elements are needed in constructing a metallic temperature transducer in order to obtain a resistance change of a practical magnitude.

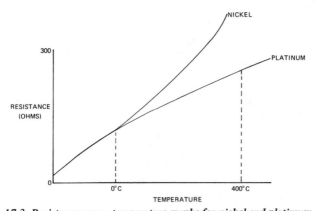

Fig. 17-3: Resistance versus temperature graphs for nickel and platinum wires

Among metallic thermoresistive transducers, the platinum/platinum-rhodium type is by far the most accurate (and most expensive) while nickel resistance transducers are more practical and economical. Metallic sensors, in addition to being the overall most accurate type of temperature transducers, have a fast response but are somewhat large and subject to mechanical damage.

The large size of metallic resistance temperature transducers makes them impractical for measuring localized temperature; consequently they find wider application in analytical instruments than in physiological monitoring devices (in gas chromatography, for example, they are sometimes used as thermal conductivity detectors).

B. Semiconductor Temperature Transducers

Semiconductor temperature sensing devices can be either solid crystal *temperature-resistive devices* or miniature semiconductor junction diodes. Generally both types have negative temperature coefficients, some exhibiting as much as a 10 percent change in resistance per degree centigrade. Figure 17-4 shows a simple temperature-resistance curve for a semiconductor temperature transducer. Note that although the response is large it is not too linear. Even so, due to their very small size, semiconductor temperature transducers are widely used to measure localized temperature changes where the use of metallic transducers would be virtually impossible.

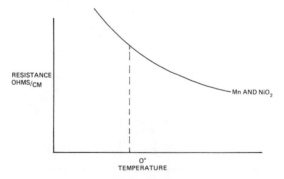

Fig. 17-4: Relative resistance versus temperature curve of a semiconductor temperature transducer of manganese and nickel oxide

The commonest form of semiconductor temperature transducers are **thermistors,** which are compounds of metallic oxides compressed into beads or discs under high pressure and temperature (Figure 17-5). The signal characteristics of these elements are, in many instances, nonlinear, but this drawback is acceptable in the light of their high sensitivity and output. They are also rugged and small, have fast response times, and are cheaper than metallic temperature transducers.

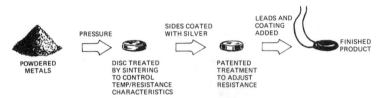

Fig. 17-5: Precision thermistor manufacturing process (courtesy of Yellow Springs Instrument Co., Yellow Springs, Ohio 45387, USA)

Silicon semiconductor junction diodes as described in Chapter 12 can be employed as temperature-sensing transducers, based on the fact that as the temperature of a *P-N* junction increases, leakage current also increases. Since voltage is the product of the resistance times the current ($E = I \times R$), if a *constant current* from an external source is maintained through the junction, temperature variations will result in proportional voltage changes, which are a function of the junction temperature. Inexpensive silicon diodes can easily be used as temperature transducers within normal temperature ranges by placing the sensing diode in one leg of a Wheatstone bridge circuit and calibrating the bridge by exposure to known temperatures.

Thermocouples

Thermocouple transducers are based on the principle that if two dissimilar metal strips (or wires) are joined at one end (the temperature junction), a potential difference which is a function of the temperature at the contact point will result between the other two ends. To use this property to measure temperature, it is necessary to have two junctions: one at the unknown temperature and one kept at a known reference temperature. Figure 17-6 shows how a thermocouple transducer can be used to measure the temperature difference between two points, P_1 and P_2, having temperatures T_1 and T_2. P_1 serves as the reference junction and is usually kept at a constant known temperature (*eg*, 0°C in an ice bath).

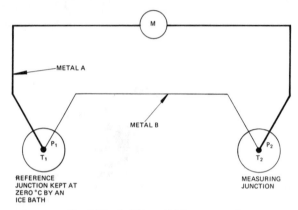

Fig. 17-6: A differential thermocouple

Some common types of thermocouples are made of copper-constantan, iron-constantan, tungsten-rhenium, and chromel-alumel. A temperature-sensitive junction can be made by soldering, welding, or even twisting two dissimilar metal wires together, but care must be taken not to cause excessive mechanical damage to the wires because permanent output errors can result due to the formation of temperature gradients and parasitic voltages at damaged points.

Thermocouples are advantageous in that they are accurate, small, and have fast response times. They exhibit marked disadvantage in that they must be used in conjunction with a reference (cold) junction (*ie*, they measure relative and not absolute temperatures. In addition to requiring a reference junction, the output response of a thermocouple is small when compared with that of a thermistor (approximately 5 mv/°C for thermistors). However, for nonprecision work their simplified construction and stability make them extremely popular. Table 17-1 lists the relative advantages and disadvantages of various types of temperature transducers. Some applications of thermocouples are in the measurement of physiological temperatures, such as skin, intramuscular, and intracranial pressures.

TABLE 17-1

RELATIVE MERITS OF THREE TYPES OF
THERMOELECTRIC TRANSDUCERS

TYPE	LINEARITY	ADVANTAGES	DISADVANTAGES
Metallic-resistance	Excellent	Stable High output Fast response	Subject to mechanical damage Expensive Chemically unstable
Thermistor	Poor	Small Rugged Chemically inert Excellent sensitivity High output	Requires aging Nonlinear
Thermocouple	Good	Small Fast response	Requires reference junction Chemically unstable

CHEMOELECTRIC TRANSDUCERS

To a physician, the measurement of blood gas levels (pCO_2 pO_2), blood pH, and the blood's circulating ionic elements is of prime importance in evaluating the status of an individual's health. In order to measure any one of these parameters, a transducer, capable of transforming chemical activity or concentration into a proportional electrical quantity, is required.

The commonest chemoelectric transducer in use is the **pH electrode**. Used in conjunction with a standard reference electrode, the pH electrode measures the concentration (or more correctly the activity) of hydrogen ion in an unknown solution. To understand how this is accomplished, and in turn to simplify the understanding of pO_2 and pCO_2 gas transducers, requires some knowledge of *half cell* or *electrode potentials*. Let us briefly review how electrode potentials are developed.

When a metal is immersed in an electrolyte solution of its own ions, two opposing reactions take place that result in a potential being developed across the metal-solution interface. In Figure

17-7, (1) metallic ions pass *into* solution, and (2) metallic ions pass *out* of the solution. When equilibrium is reached, two charge layers of opposite potential result at the interface. The polarity of these charge layers (inner and outer) is such that positive ions gather in the liquid phase in contact with the electrode, while electrons build up a negative layer on the metal surface. The magnitude of the layers is controlled by (a) how easily the metal gives up ions to the solution, and (b) the concentration of metal ions already in solution. The difference in potential produced across the interface is referred to as the **half cell** or **electrode potential.**

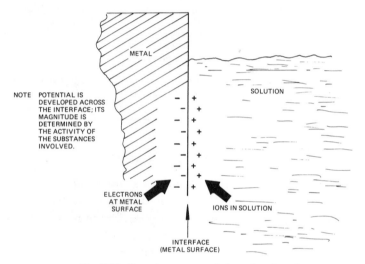

Fig. 17-7: Reaction at a metal-electrolyte interface

Measurement of a single, absolute, electrode potential is obviously impossible, for in order to detect the voltage, a second electrode must be placed into the electrolyte, thereby creating a second (its own) electrode potential. As a solution to this problem, the hydrogen gas electrode was chosen as a (zero potential) standard reference and all other electrodes are compared to it. (Two other common and somewhat more practical reference electrodes are calomel ($Hg\text{-}Hg_2\text{-}Cl_2$) and silver ($Ag\text{-}AgCl$) electrodes).

In the measurement of pH one of these reference electrodes is used in conjunction with a glass electrode to produce a *glass electrode assembly.* The glass electrode is the primary transducer and its operation is illustrated in Figure 17-8. A special type of glass when used as the interface separating two solutions, (*A*) and (*B*), of different hydrogen ion concentration shows a potential difference between its two surfaces. The magnitude of the potential is a function of the *difference* in hydrogen ion concentration between the two solutions. By placing a solution with a known hydrogen ion concentration on one side of the glass, the pH of an unknown solution of the other side can indirectly be determined.

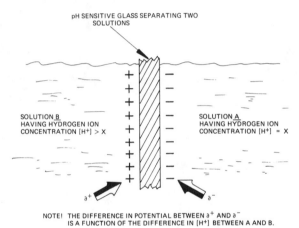

pH SENSITIVE GLASS SEPARATING TWO
SOLUTIONS

SOLUTION B
HAVING HYDROGEN ION
CONCENTRATION [H+] > X

SOLUTION A
HAVING HYDROGEN ION
CONCENTRATION [H+] = X

a^+ a^-

NOTE! THE DIFFERENCE IN POTENTIAL BETWEEN a^+ AND a^-
IS A FUNCTION OF THE DIFFERENCE IN [H+] BETWEEN A AND B.

Fig. 17-8: Simplified diagram of the action of pH sensitive glass

Figure 17-9 demonstrates the construction of a typical glass pH electrode assembly. At (1), an internal metal reference electrode is immersed in a solution of known hydrogen ion concentration. Since a metal/solution interface is created, a potential (E_1) results at the metal surface. At (2), the known electrolyte solution and reference electrode are then sealed within a pH-sensitive glass envelope or bulb. At (3), when the bulb is immersed in a solution having a different hydrogen ion concentration from that of the known electrolyte, a potential difference (E_2) develops across the glass interface. This voltage is reflected through the known electrolyte solution causing a change in the potential of E_1 (Δ

E_1). At (4), when an external reference electrode (whose potential (E_0) is designated by convention as zero is *also* immersed in the unknown solution, the resulting potential difference E_{pH} between E_0 and E_1 is a function of the hydrogen ion concentration in the unknown solution, and can be measured by use of an appropriate high input impedance voltmeter. To determine the pH, the voltage can then be compared to potentials produced by known standard

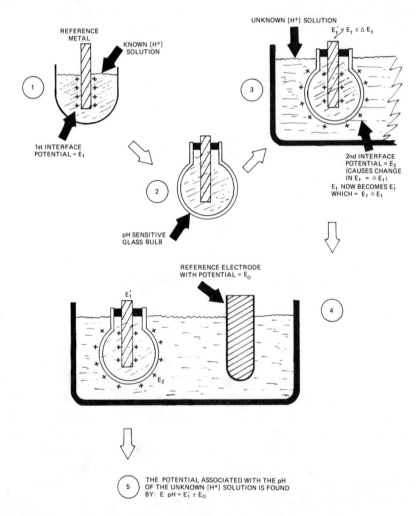

Fig. 17-9: Steps in the preparation of a pH electrode assembly and pH determination

pH solutions. In a typical pH meter, this is accomplished by adjustment and calibration of the meter scale with known pH solutions, prior to use.

The foregoing "simplified" discussion is ample evidence that the theory behind chemoelectric transducers is far from simple. The fundamental concepts involved fall into the realm of physical chemistry. However, an elementary understanding of their operation can be helpful in many areas of medical electronics.

The one important fact that comes to light in discussing pH measurement is that there is no such thing as a *simple* chemoelectric transducer; all of them involve interactions between numerous different phases and the resulting interface potentials. The study of dissolved gases in physiological fluids further complicates an already difficult problem by adding yet another phase and consequently another interface.

To measure the concentration of a gas in physiological fluid (blood, tissue, etc) requires that either (a) the transducer be highly selective or (b) the gas first be separated from the fluid and then measured. The latter method introduces the possibility of error due to loss of the gas; consequently, the ideal method seems to be measurement by use of a selective transducer.

In the measurement of fluid pH, a set of two chemoelectric transducers is placed directly into the solution in question (a reference and a measuring electrode) and the concentration of hydrogen ion is measured directly. With gases the problem is a little more difficult. No simple devices selective for pO_2 or pCO_2 are available that will measure the concentrations of these substances directly; however, this problem can be solved in one of the following two ways: Two transducers (or electrodes) are placed in a captive electrolyte solution. The electrolyte and the two electrodes are then sealed within a selectively permeable membrane that will only pass the gas in question (O_2 or CO_2). The gas, after crossing the membrane can (1) react directly with one of the electrodes, producing a potential proportional to concentration, or (2) it can react with the captive electrolyte solution, causing a pH change which is detected by a pH electrode. The pH change then becomes an indirect indicator of the concentration of the gas. Figure 17-10 shows diagramatically the two systems. Note that in the CO_2 sensing system, one of the electrodes is a pH electrode, while in the other system it is an electrode reactive to oxygen.

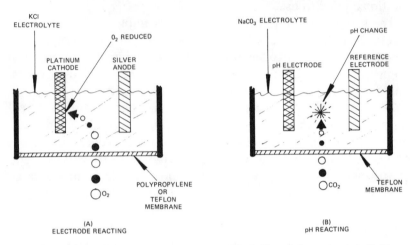

Fig. 17-10: pO_2 and pCO_2 gas electrodes - simplified. (from information supplied by
Beckman Instruments, Fullerton, California)

In recent years electrodes that are sensitive to a single ionic species, as pH electrodes are, have been developed. These chemoelectric transducers are called **specific ion electrodes.** Electrodes selective for monovalent (Cl^-, Na^+, etc) ions as well as some divalent ions (Ca^{++}, Mg^{++}) have been developed and, although problems with sensitivity and application procedures were common when they were first introduced, the effects of these problems are gradually being reduced and specific ion electrodes are becoming more and more popular.

PHOTOELECTRIC TRANSDUCERS

Probably the singly most important transducer found in instruments today is the **optical** (or **photoelectric**) **transducer.** These invaluable devices fall into two general classes: (1) *tube type photoelectric transducers,* and (2) *semiconductor photoelectric transducers;* and both types of phototransducers can be further divided into subgroups.

Tube type photoelectric transducers may be (a) **photodiodes,** which in turn may be (1) *vacuum* or (2) *gas-filled;* or they may be

(b) **photomultipliers,** which may be (1) *circular,* (2) *linear,* (3) *box,* or (4) *venetian blind.*

Semiconductor photoelectric transducers may be (a) **photocells,** which may be (1) *photoconductive,* (2) *photovoltaic* (barrier layer), or (3) *avalanche photodiodes;* or they may be (b) **phototransistors.**

All photoelectric transducers function due to the phenomenon known as the *photoelectric effect.* Photoelectric action can be summarized by saying that some materials (namely metals and alkali metals) when exposed to radiation emit or release electrons (referred to as **photoelectrons**). In tube type photoelectric transducers, the photoelectrons emitted pass from the metal surface into a gas or vacuum, while in semiconductor photoelectric transducers the electrons are excited into a current-carrying state *within* the solid material.

Some characteristics of photoemissive materials should be emphasized. The first is **excitation frequency** (f_{ex}). Every material has its own excitation frequency, and light waves, no matter how intense, of a frequency lower than f_{ex} will *not* cause photoemission. The second characteristic concerns **response.** The number of photoelectrons emitted by a substance (measured as circuit current flow) is directly proportional to the light intensity (once f_{ex} has been exceeded). It is these two characteristics of the photoelectric effect that make photoelectric transducers invaluable in many medical instruments, such as colorimeters and spectrophotometers, to name just two.

Phototubes

Phototubes of either the vacuum or gas-filled variety consist of a photosensitive cathode (or emitter) and a positive anode, both sealed into a glass envelope. The cathode is a curved piece of metal coated with a photosensitive material (common coatings in general use are the cesium-antimony and multi-alkali (Sb/K/Na/Cs) types). When light strikes the photocathode, electrons are emitted and attracted to the positive anode, producing current flow in the external circuit. Figure 17-11 shows a diagram of a basic photodiode. The major difference between gas and vacuum photodiodes is that the former contain an inert gas which is ionized by the impact of photoelectrons from the cathode and therefore causes amplification of the primary photocurrent. Gas photodiodes have poorer stability and shorter lives than vacuum photodiodes, but their increased sensitivity is obtained at small expense (the gas) and as a result they are widely used.

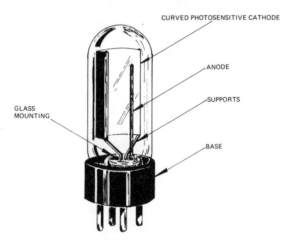

Fig. 17-11: A simplified phototube (photodiode)

An important characteristic of every photodiode is its spectral response: at what wave length does the tube exhibit its highest sensitivity? In analytical instrumentation it is this characteristic that determines the type of light source, filters, etc, that are to be used with any chosen transducer. Spectral response is usually given by the manufacturer as an *s* number (*s-1*, *s-2*, etc.) which identifies its sensitivity at a specific wave length.

Additional characteristics also important when selecting a photoelectric transducer for a particular application or even substitution of another can be found at the end of this section.

Photomultipliers

The poor sensitivity and limited frequency response of a photo tube become limiting factors in applications in which low-intensity, rapidly changing light levels are to be detected. The amount of photocurrent produced in such applications is so small that high-gain amplifiers must be used before a practical amplitude is achieved. When a standard amplifier is utilized for this purpose, it amplifies not only the primary photocurrent but also any electrical noise produced in generating that current; therefore, the resulting output exhibits a high noise level as well as a high signal level. Put another way, the system has a low signal-to-noise ratio. To overcome this difficulty the amplifying phototube or **photomultiplier** was developed. Photomultipliers combine the effects of *photoemission* and *secondary emission* to amplify low level light signals to the extent that gains of 10^6 or 10^7 are practical.

In a conventional phototube the two active elements are the *photocathode* and the *anode*. A third element found in photomultipliers is the **dynode** and there are from 10 to 14 dynodes in a typical photomultiplier, depending upon its design. Photocurrent produced in a conventional photodiode flows from cathode directly to the anode, but in photomultipliers there is a different action (Figure 17-12). Primary photoelectrons produced by striking the photocathode are attracted to the *first* dynode (due to its location and positive potential). Upon impact at the dynode a single high-energy photoelectron causes secondary emission of several lower energy electrons. When emitted, these secondary electrons are attracted by the *second* dynode (since it is held at a positive voltage with respect to dynode number one) and the same process of secondary emission occurs again. Since one primary electron can yield from three to six secondary electrons, the reason for the name *photomultiplier* becomes obvious; the dynode

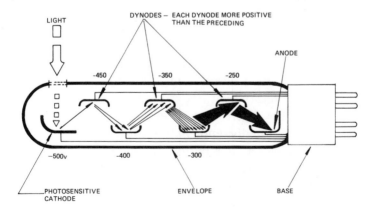

Fig. 17-12: Pictorial diagram of a typical photomultiplier

action is repeated 10 to 14 times. Some photomultipliers contain other elements such as accelerating grids or focusing plates, but their overall operation is basically the same.

Dynode configurations in photomultipliers are the result of different applications and variation in required characteristics. The first design developed was the *circular cage photomultiplier* consisting of a photocathode, nine curved dynodes in a circular arrangement, and the anode. A second design commercially available is the *linear photomultiplier* of which there is more than one form. *Box type* and *venetian blind* dynode configurations are not quite as responsive as the previous two due to the effects of electron transit-time dispersion between dynodes that results in loss of gain. (Transit-time dispersion refers to the by-passing or skipping of dynodes by electrons due to the tendency of the electron stream to "fan out" as it gets farther from its point of origin.) Generally, the longer the transit-time (dynode to dynode), the greater will be the dispersion unless it is compensated for by focusing elements or dynode configuration.

Each successive dynode in a photomultiplier requires an operating voltage greater than that of the preceding one. Voltage divider networks are used to supply these operating potentials.

Within limits, the gain and sensitivity of a photomultiplier can be controlled by the applied dynode voltages. An increase in dynode voltage usually produces an increase in gain up to a certain point, but beyond this point no further gain, and at times even a decrease in gain, can occur.

Two practical points that should be emphasized concerning the use of photomultipliers are (1) fatigue and (2) low temperature operation. In the case of fatigue (loss of photocathode sensitivity), the effect can be either absolute or temporary. When exposed to unusually high intensity light, the cathode emits photoelectrons at a high rate, thereby decreasing its sensitivity. (Electrons emitted are not replaced rapidly enough by the cathode circuit.) The cathode may recover after a period of time stored in darkness or the effect may be permanent, depending on the length and intensity of the exposure to light. For this reason photomultipliers found in analytical instruments should *never* have their protective covers removed while power is applied to them.

The second practical point to consider in relation to photo-multipliers is their operation at low temperatures (especially in places of high humidity). Since the light levels or changes in intensity detected by these devices are at times very low, any interference in the optical path will result in an inaccurate response. Low temperature (and high humidity) environments that permit condensation to occur upon the glass windows of photo-multipliers will therefore result in false output signals.

Although both phototubes and photomultipliers generate un-desirable electrical noise due to both (a) *thermonic emission,* and (b) *shot noise,* (caused by photo and secondary emission), photomultipliers decrease the overall effects of thermonic emis-sion; therefore, the signal-to-noise ratio of a photomultiplier is much superior to that of a conventional photodiode. To obtain maximum efficiency from both types of phototubes the following conditions should be observed:

1. Never store phototubes in light, or at high temperatures.
2. Do not use them, if at all possible, in high temperature or high humidity environments, or in areas producing prolonged vibration or shock effects.
3. Never exceed the maximum prescribed voltage ratings.

Semiconductor Photo-Transducers

Three materials used in the production of semiconductor devices, selenium, germanium and silicon, exhibit a high variation in conductivity when exposed to light. (This is also true of some metal sulfides.) This property of photo-mediated conducting is utilized in producing semiconductor phototransducers. These devices can be divided into two general groups: (1) **photocells** and (2) **phototransistors.**

Photocells come in two forms: (1) *photo-conductive* cells and (2) *photovoltaic* (or *photogalvanic*) cells. Photoconductive cells consist of an inert support medium (usually glass or ceramic in nature) upon which a thin layer of photosensitive material is deposited. Two electrodes are connected to the end points of the photosensitive ribbon. When placed in a circuit, the device acts like a resistor that is sensitive to changes in light intensity. By

convention the prime characteristic of the cell is defined not as its
resistance change, but as its *increase in conductivity when exposed
to increased light intensity.* Due to their low cost and versatility
cadmium sulfide photoconductive cells (Figure 17-13) are probably the most widely utilized phototransducers in general use.
They are used in computer control circuits as well as in some
special-application analytical instruments (Calbiometer®). Note
that all photoconductive cells are *passive* transducers.

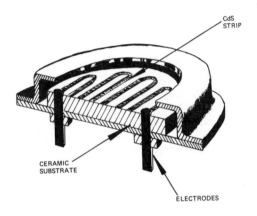

CdS
STRIP

CERAMIC
SUBSTRATE

ELECTRODES

Fig. 17-13: A cadmium sulfide photoconductive cell

An example of an *active* photo-transducer is the photovoltaic
cell which can take one of three forms. It can either be (1) a *barrier
layer* type, (2) a *junction* device, or (3) a *point contact diode.*

Barrier layer cells were the first type of photovoltaic cell to be
developed. In their construction (Figure 17-14) a metal support
medium is formed (which also acts as one terminal of the voltaic
cell) upon which a covering film of semiconductive material is laid.
A transparent film of metal is then sprayed over the semiconduct-
ing layer to act as the other terminal. The semiconductor layers
commonly used are selenium or cuprous oxide. When light strikes
the photosensitive layer, electrons are generated and pass into the
transparent metal layer, producing a potential difference between
the cell terminals. This voltage can then be used to drive a
galvanometer or some other detection device.

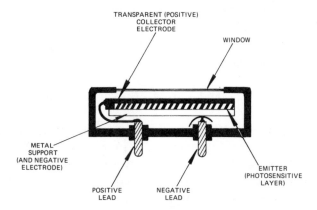

Fig. 17-14: Simplified diagram of a barrier layer cell

Junction photocells employ two types of semiconductive material, formed into a junction diode and held in a plastic support medium. They are unique in that they may be used in one of two ways: (1) as a *photoconductive* transducer, or (2) as a *photovoltaic* transducer. Use as a **photoconductive transducer** calls for reverse biasing the diode and focusing the light to be detected upon its junction. Variations in load current occur when the intensity of the light incident upon the junction changes; consequently, it is functioning as a photoconductive transducer (Figure 17-15).

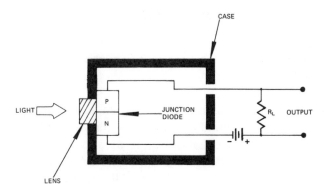

Fig. 17-15:   A junction photodiode (Note: lens is focused onto the junction.) Reproduced by permission of the Department of the Army.

When connected into a circuit *without* a power source, the above described cell becomes a **photovoltaic cell,** converting radiant energy directly into electrical current. Light striking the junction produces electron-hole pairs with sufficient energy to overcome the potential gradient produced when the junction was formed (Chapter 12) and current flow results in the external circuit.

The materials commonly used in the manufacture of junction photo-transducers are germanium (*PN* junction) and silicon (used for solar cells) *N* on *P* or *P* on *N*. Figure 17-16 shows a germanium **point contact photodiode;** since it requires an external power source to operate, it is also considered as a photoconductive device. Normally there is a high resistance to current flow from the germanium wafer to the metal whisker due to reverse biasing but, when focused light strikes the wafer in the region of the junction, this bias is overcome and conduction occurs.

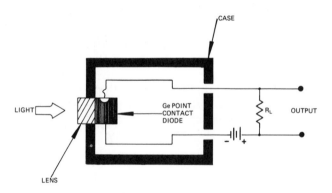

Fig. 17-16: *A germanium point contact photodiode. Reproduced by permission of the Department of the Army.*

The discovery of a phenomenon known as **avalanche effect** (a type of intracrystal secondary emission) has led to the development by Bell Telephone Laboratories of photodiodes that have built-in amplification. Where standard photodiodes produce one photoelectron per photon of incident light, some experimental diodes can produce up to 250 electrons per photon. These devices are referred to as **avalanche photodiodes.** Figure 17-17 shows an

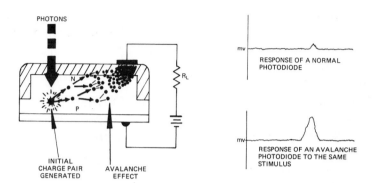

Fig. 17-17: An avalanche photodiode

avalanche photodiode and its response to a weak light pulse, as compared to a conventional photodiode.

Photo-Transistors

By constructing two *PN* junction photodiodes back-to-back, a **phototransistor** can be formed. The base of the transistor is the photosensitive region. If normal transistor bias is applied to both junctions, light changes focused on the base result in collector potential changes which are highly amplified reproductions of those at the base (Figure 17-18). Phototransistors exhibit a gain of 50 to 500 times that found in photodiodes.

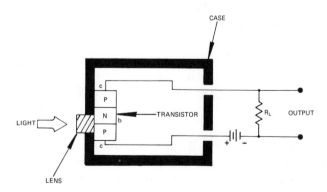

Fig. 17-18: A phototransistor (Note: lens is focused on the emitter-base junction.)
Reproduced by permission of the Department of the Army.

The advantages of semiconductor photodetectors are similar to those of semiconductors in general when compared to conventionally sized vacuum tube devices: small size, low operating voltages, low power consumption and low noise levels, as well as high efficiency and unsophisticated circuitry.

Some important factors that should be considered when determining the particular application of a photo transducer are:

1. Spectral response (wave length *vs.* output)
2. Linearity (intensity *vs* output)
3. Frequency response
4. Noise level (signal-to-noise ratio)
5. Interference (temperature, vibration, energy)
6. Dark current values
7. Transit-time (cathode to anode or dynode)
8. Dynode properties
9. Dynode configuration } photomultipliers only
10. Gain characteristics

Items 1 through 6 are especially important in analytical instrument applications.

NUCLEAR TRANSDUCERS
RADIOACTIVE ENERGY TRANSDUCERS

Radioactive energy transducers will not be discussed in great detail since their study truly belongs in the realm of nuclear chemistry and physics. A description of three common types should suffice to give an adequate understanding of the basic principles used in their design. First, let us take a quick look at the common forms of nuclear energy.

In measurement of nuclear activity (or radioactivity as it is commonly referred to), the four most mentioned types are:

The **alpha particle** (a): a helium nucleus;

The **beta particle** (β): A high velocity electron-like particle;

The **gamma ray** (σ): Wave-like energy having no mass;

The **x-ray** (X): Also wavelike without mass;

The properties of radiation most often used in measuring its effect are: (1) penetrating ability, (2) reflectability, and (3) ionizing ability.

Of the four types of radiation, the three most often encountered in medical applications are the *beta, gamma,* and *x-ray* forms.
The extensive use of these energy types is a result of their much
higher penetrating ability when compared to the alpha particle
(Figure 17-19). For example, a sheet of paper is capable of
preventing alpha particle passage, but not even lead or concrete
will stop gamma penetration completely. How is such high energy
radiation produced and how do its various forms differ? Let us
take a minute to determine this.

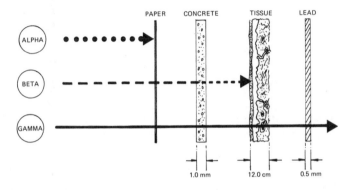

*Fig. 17-19:   Relative penetrating power of radioactive particles. (1 million electron volt
            source)*

A phenomenon utilized in photomultiplier tubes called *secondary emission* is the result of a relatively high energy electron
striking a substance and causing the release of other "secondary"
electrons from the outer orbit of an atom. If the primary electron
is of a high enough velocity (energy content), it penetrates deep
into the structure of the atom, causing the subsequent release of
high energy electrons and waves of photons called **x-rays.** Further
increasing the energy of the invading primary particle to the point
that it is capable of producing nuclear disintegration results in the
release of even higher energy photons called **gamma rays.** In
addition to gamma rays, nuclear disintegration can also generate a
high velocity, negatively charged particle with the mass of an
electron called a **beta particle.** Should the substance under
bombardment happen to be helium gas, and if particle bombard-

ment causes the ejection of two electrons, the species remaining is an **alpha particle** (a helium nucleus consisting of two protons and two neutrons). This process is diagrammed in Figure 17-20.

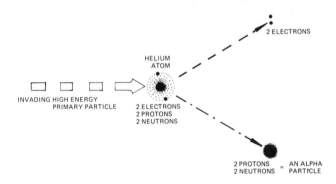

Fig. 17-20: Alpha particle generation by nuclear disintegration

The above example shows that different types of "artificial" or induced radiation can be produced by bombardment of an atom with high velocity particles; in addition, many chemical elements have naturally radioactive forms called **radioisotopes.** Isotopes are atoms of a particular element with different masses due to different numbers of protons and neutrons.

The primary effect of radiation is *ionization:* the production of electron-positive ion pairs within the medium the radiation strikes. For this reason all transducers used to detect radiation can be classified as **ionization transducers.** Some function by measuring the number of ion pairs produced, while others detect the number of individual rays; both types are described in the following paragraphs.

The **ionization chamber** is one example of a transducer used for the detection of ionizing radiation. It consists of two electrodes maintained at a potential difference by an external voltage source within a gas-filled chamber. The chamber has an entrance window through which the radiation enters (Figure 17-21). Ionizing radiation entering the chamber causes ion pair production by displacing an orbital electron from an atom. The electrodes attract the charged particles, resulting in a potential change at each electrode that is proportional to the number of ion pairs produced. This, in effect, measures the quantity of *radiant energy per unit time.*

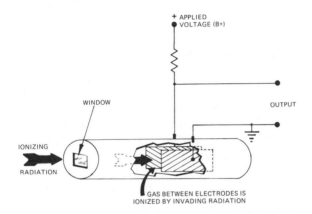

Fig. 17-21: A simplified diagram of an ionization chamber

The avalanche effect that high velocity electrons are capable of producing (electrons released by *radiation* ionization produce other charge pairs by *impact* ionization) makes gas-filled ionization detectors adaptable—with appropriate changes in chamber design, applied voltage, and gas composition—as **counting chambers.** Counting chambers can be either (a) proportional counters or (b) Geiger counters, depending upon the magnitude of the potential applied to the electrodes. At low potentials (below 500 volts) the ionization chamber functions as a detector of primary ionizations as noted in the preceding paragraph where the *output is directly proportional to the number of ions formed.* (No avalanche ionization takes place). When the voltage is increased to between 500 and 750 volts, the ionization chamber (with correct gas composition, etc.) becomes a **proportional counter.** Due to the higher potential, ionized electron velocity increases and a controlled process of avalanche ionization results; the output signal then becomes a function of the *energy dissipated by the incident particle,* making it possible to discriminate between relatively low energy alpha particles and higher energy beta particles. These transducers are also sensitive to gamma radiation. By the addition of an argon/alcohol gas mixture and an increase in operating voltage to a value in excess of 1,000 volts, we obtain a detector that functions as an individual particle counter whose output pulses are of a constant amplitude regardless of incident energy. The number of pulses, however, is a direct count of the number of incident particles that produce ionization. This type of ionization detector is called a **Geiger Muller counter** (commonly referred to as simply Geiger counter).

Another common radiation detector used extensively in medicine is the **scintillation counter**. The detector used in these instruments is really a combination of two transducers: (1) a radioactive-to-optical energy converter, and (2) an optical-to-electrical energy converter. The radioactive-to-optical transducer can be a crystal (of potassium or sodium iodide) or a phosphor-coated screen. When struck by radiation the phosphor or crystal transforms the radiation into flashes of light. In the optical-to-electrical transducer, coupling a photomultiplier to the crystal (or screen) causes the light flashes to yield electrical output pulses (Figure 17-22).

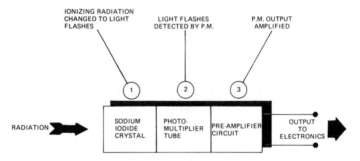

Fig. 17-22: Block diagram of a scintillation detector

Semiconductor radiation detectors recently developed show improved efficiency over gas detectors and this fact coupled with their small size is contributing to their increasing utilization, predominantly in nuclear spectroscopy. An example of such a **solid state ionization detector** is a **crystal counter**. These detectors are made of a nonconducting crystal (diamond, silver chloride, or silver bromide) that has been doped with silicon or germanium to decrease dark-current effects. When radiation strikes a crystal that has been placed into a circuit containing a load resistor and voltage source, ionic pairs are produced within its structure, causing a pulse of current that can be detected at the load resistor. The crystal acts somewhat like a switch that is sensitive to radiation. Other types of semiconductor ionization detectors are: (1) surface-junction detectors, (2) surface-barrier detectors, (3) lithium-ion drift detectors, and (4) radiation-induced photoconductivity detectors.

NOTE: All ionization detectors are passive transducers.

FLOW RATE TRANSDUCERS

The simplest method of measuring the rate at which a fluid is flowing through a closed system is to insert a rotating (vane) displacement meter into the stream and count the number of revolutions per unit time. Comparing this value to standardized or calibrated values yields the unknown flow rate. Such a direct measurement method is quite adequate for nonliving systems, but how does one insert a relatively large displacement meter into a human artery without affecting or disrupting the system's function? Although this method has been used in the past, the answer is, today one doesn't. The measurement of fluid flow in humans primarily involves blood and, since the ideal clinical technique calls for noninvasive methods, more sophisticated and indirect techniques are required. Blood flow is measured with detectors ranging from radiation detectors to thermal conductivity probes and electromagnetic flow meters.

The most common transducers used in blood flow analysis today are: (1) **electromagnetic detectors**, (2) **thermal detectors**, (3) **sonic detectors**, and (4) **ionization detectors**. In each case, the transducer employed is measuring flow rate by an *indirect* method that is dependent upon some detectable phenomenon produced as a result of the flow. Rather than discussing the individual transducers involved, this section deals instead with the method in which some transducers are employed to measure blood flow rates.

Electromagnetic Detectors

The most widely used device in the measurement of blood flow is the **electromagnetic flow meter**. The transducer used in electromagnetic blood flow analysis makes use of the basic principle that a conductor moving through a magnetic field will have an EMF induced into it, the orientation of which is perpendicular to both the direction of the magnetic field and the direction of conductor motion—the same fundamental principle upon which generators function (Figure 23A). In the case of blood flow analysis, the conductor is the blood itself, although the principle can be applied to any conductive fluid. Figure 17-23B shows diagramatically the construction of a typical electromagnetic blood flow transducer. The electromagnet produces a magnetic field B which passes through the vessel within which the blood is flowing. Through the influence of the magnetic field on the moving blood, an electric field E is induced, which is perpendicular to both the direction of B and the blood flow. The electric field produces a voltage that is sensed by electrodes (E_1 and E_2), processed, and indicated on a flow meter. The magnitude of E is a function of (1) the magnetic field intensity, given by B; (2) the distance between E_1 and E_2; and (3) the fluid velocity. With the magnetic field intensity and electrode placement fixed by design, E then becomes a function of the flow rate alone and, with the device properly calibrated, a reliable indicator of the blood's instantaneous velocity.

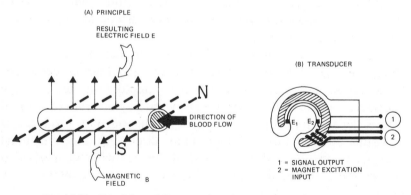

Fig. 17-23: Principle and diagram of an electromagnetic flow transducer

The excitation voltage applied to these transducers can be DC, sine wave, square wave, or even trapezoidal in form. However, AC excitation voltages are in general use because voltages that are unrelated to flow rate (called *spurious polarization potentials*) are severe in the DC type devices. More recently, pulsed AC voltages have also been found to be effective in limiting this effect.

Thermal Detectors

When a heated element is immersed in a fluid stream (gas or liquid), the amount of heat lost by the element into the moving fluid is a function of the rate at which the fluid is moving. By measuring the power required to maintain a constant temperature at the heated element, a measurement of the relative flow rate can be obtained. Flow transducers utilizing this principle are called **thermal velocity probes.** Intravascular velocity probes can take the form of heated wires, metal films, or more commonly thermistors. Inserted by catheter into the lumen of a vessel, these transducers are connected to a self-balancing DC Wheatstone bridge circuit which controls the probe temperature, keeps it constant, and records the amount of energy required to do so. A second thermister is generally used to measure the blood temperature so that the output will be insensitive to temperature changes of the blood itself.

Sonic Detectors

Recently the field of ultrasonics has found its way into the area of blood velocity determination. One popular method employs two piezo-electric transducers located a known distance apart in a fluid stream. From measurements of the time it takes pulsed ultrasound to travel the known distance in both directions, the flow rate can be calculated. This is based on the fact that the sound will travel *faster* when transmitted in the direction the blood is moving, and *slower* when transmitted in the opposite direction. These devices are known as **pulsed ultrasonic flow meters.**

A second acoustic method of blood flow rate determination incorporates use of the **Doppler effect.** Put simply, the Doppler principle states that if the transmitting source and the receiver of a sound wave are *both stationary,* then the frequency of the received signal is the *same* as the frequency of the transmitted signal, *but* if *either* the source or the receiver are *moving* toward or away from each other, the received frequency will differ from the true transmitted frequency, such that it will be *higher for approach* and *lower for separation* (Figure 17-24*A*). The difference between the two frequencies is known as the **Doppler shift** and its magnitude can be used to determine the velocity of the moving element. When a stationary piezo-electric transducer is placed in such a position that it focuses a pulse of ultrasound into the lumen of a vessel, the moving blood particles reflect the signal

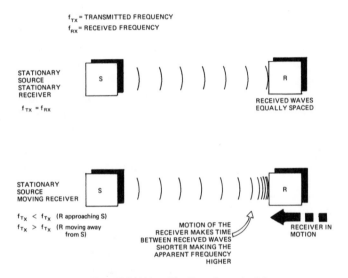

Fig. 17-24(A):   The Doppler principle

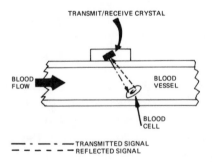

Fig. 17-24(B): Simplified diagram of a Doppler blood flow transducer so that the frequency difference between the transmitted pulse and the received pulse is a function of the velocity of the reflecting particles—and hence a relative indicator of flow rate. This phenomenon has led to the development of numerous ultrasonic transducers, some of which are placed directly around the vessel (Figure 17-24*B*), as well as those transducers that can transmit and receive through layers of tissue.

Ionization Detectors

Ionization detectors, primarily **scintillation counters,** are used in dilution techniques that employ radioisotope tracers for flow rate analysis. A known amount of radioactive material (usually a gamma source) is injected into the patient and an ionization detector is focused over a specified vessel. Since the injected particles are distributed throughout the blood in a definite pattern due to blood flow past the injection point, a curve such as that shown in Figure 17-25 results when the intensity of the detected radiation is plotted against time. The area under the curve is a function of the vessel's response to the sudden injection and consequently also a function of the flow rate.

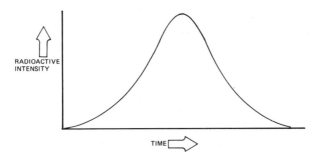

Fig. 17-25: Radioactive tracer dilution curve (used for flow rate analysis)

Another dilution technique involves the same rate-dependent distribution theory as the radioisotope tracer method, but injection of a nontoxic dye into the vascular system replaces the isotope injection. An optical transducer detects density changes in blood flowing through a cuvette via a cannula (note that this is an invasion technique) and the result is a curve similar to that in

Figure 17-25, but relating density to time instead of radioactivity to time.

Although each of these types of flow transducers have been used in various applications, as noted previously the most widely used type is the electromagnetic flow transducer, followed by the ultrasonic type. More detailed information concerning the other types of transducers can be found in the references given for this chapter.

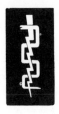

a primer on understanding instruments

CHAPTER 18

A vast amount of electronic instrumentation found in today's modern hospitals is greatly diversified in function and application. Nevertheless, any device that operates electronically consists of networks or systems that are adaptations of one or more basic circuits. These circuits in turn are constructed in various ways from a limited number of—in fact, just six—fundamental types of components. With the correct approach and familiarity with these (1) basic circuits and (2) components, as well as (3) a little knowledge of terminology, electronic instrumentation, whatever its function, design, or application, becomes much easier to understand.

The six basic elements or components that make up virtually all electronic devices were given in a previous chapter, but should be repeated:

1. Resistors
2. Capacitors (condensers) } The passive elements
3. Inductors (coils, chokes, transformers)

4. Vacuum tubes
5. Semiconductors } The active elements
6. Solid state or integrated circuits

These components constitute (in most cases) the sum total of all the passive and active elements that are generally found in any electronic instrument. Being able to recognize these components is an important factor in developing a proficiency for working with, and maintaining, instrumentation. Illustrations of typical elements found in electronic devices are shown on the following pages.

A biomedical instrument is only valuable when its user understands its operational capabilities and limitations, and is able

197

to recognize any deviation from normal operation; therefore, he needs some understanding of the circuits that make up the instrument. To those who are unfamiliar with instrumentation, the following paragraphs should prove helpful. The information included in them is meant to provide a clearer understanding of common terminology, circuitry and systems approach used in instrumentation.

THE OBJECTIVES OF INSTRUMENTATION

Any activity in which man involves himself has a definite pattern which can be envisioned in most cases as a cause-effect relationship. Although at certain times it may seem otherwise, everything we do (*effect*) has a reason (*cause*). A pattern that becomes most obvious in a majority of cases involves the processes of: (1) observation, by our senses; (2) communication, by our nervous system; (3) evaluation, by our brain; and (4) response, by our muscles, bones, etc.

Since one of the prime purposes of any instrument is to extend the range and/or sensitivity of man's faculties, it is quite reasonable to assume that he should design the same "systems process" into these devices as he himself uses.

A useful instrument, therefore, must meet one or more of the following requirements:

1. It should extend man's *senses* so that he is capable of detecting phenomena beyond the range or sensitivity of his normal faculties.
2. It should increase the *speed* at which he is capable of performing a particular function.
3. It should give him the capability of performing more than one function *simultaneously*.
4. It should enable him to accomplish all of the above reliably, and with *reproducibility*.
5. It should accomplish all these things *economically*.

These items constitute the basic objectives or requirements that engineers attempt to design, and users hope to obtain, in any given instrument. Because of this, instruments can be evaluated as adequate or not by an examination of their performance characteristics, which are based on these five criteria. The items most commonly used to describe an instrument's performance are given in the following paragraphs.

Since the first objective of instrumentation is to increase man's sensitivity, the first characteristic of an instrument to be considered is obvious: **sensitivity.** Sensitivity refers to the relationship between the input and the output of some device or system. A very highly sensitive instrument is one that gives a usable output when the input signal is very small.

The numerical quantities used to specify sensitivity are of several different sorts depending on the particular applications involved. The sensitivity of a meter is often given as the signal required for full-scale deflection, but in other applications, sensitivity may be given as read-out deflection or response of some other sort per unit input. Each method of specifying sensitivity has its own characteristic units. For example, in the case of temperature measurement, a transducer may yield an output voltage change of 4 mv per degree of temperature change; its sensitivity is therefore given in terms of *millivolts per degree.* A meter used for blood pressure determination may yield a read-out meter deflection of 2 divisions per mm of Hg; hence its sensitivity is given in *scale divisions per millimeter of mercury.* Whatever the units used or the way in which sensitivity is expressed, it is basically nothing more than an indication of an instrument's characteristic response to a given input stimulus.

During the evolutionary process of a successful instrument's development, design changes or improvements in one of its operating specifications invariably affect other characteristics. For example, if an instrument's sensitivity is increased, usually not only is the device more sensitive to the given quantity it is meant to measure (*eg,* nerve impulses) but, in addition, it will also show an increase in sensitivity to unwanted signals, such as background noise or artifact (muscle potentials, etc.).

To minimize this problem requires the incorporation into the instrument of another specification: **selectivity.** Basically, this characteristic indicates an instrument's capability to discriminate between wanted and unwanted signals. By the appropriate choice and design of transducers, and/or instrument circuitry, high levels of selectivity can be obtained. Terms such as *common-mode* *rejection ratio* (CMR) and *error band* are often used to indicate a measure of an instrument's selectivity, and are usually expressed as a figure of merit (*eg*, CMR of 50,000:1).

Another important specification required in all of today's sophisticated instrumentation is **linearity**. Linearity refers to the ability of an instrument to yield a faithful reproduction of a detected signal in its output. Whatever quantity or parameter a device is designed to respond to, that phenomenon has its own unique qualities of *amplitude* and *frequency*, and an instrument must be capable of detecting and reproducing them in a linear fashion. Although few if any instruments show linear response over the entire spectrum of signals they are capable of detecting, the upper and lower limits of linearity must at least equal or, better still, exceed those of the specific parameter to be measured.

This fact in turn results in a fourth instrument specification: **range**. Range can refer to the voltage or current limits an instrument is capable of detecting, but more often it refers to the band of frequencies the instrument can effectively span and respond to. For instance, an instrument used as part of an ECG system must be capable of responding to signals that vary from 0.1 to 100 Hz, while a device used in detecting muscle potentials should have an upper limit of 1,000 Hz.

Along with the specifications of sensitivity, selectivity, linearity and range, a good instrument must incorporate **stability** and **reliability** into its profile. Unless an instrument is capable of maintaining stable values of sensitivity, etc., its ability to furnish reliable information is questionable and it is of little value in the science of biomedical measurement and instrumentation.

All instrument users and potential users should be cognizant of the instrument specifications just summarized as applied to the particular devices with which they work. Without such knowledge, a realistic and logical evaluation of an instrument and its performance is inadequate if not impossible.

THE ELEMENTARY INSTRUMENT COMPLEX

A mechanical or electrical device can usually be described in one of three ways (1) superficially, (2) systematically, or (3) analytically. The block diagram, modular, or "systems" approach lends itself best to those interested in developing a general understanding of instrumentation. This approach can quickly be applied to almost any device one may encounter because the functional units within an instrument system are in most cases nothing more than modified and sophisticated examples of a number of basic circuits. By knowing what these basic circuits do, and mentally dividing an instrument into a few basic systems, the student can acquire a working understanding of its operation with relatively little effort.

Any instrument can be considered in a highly simplified manner as performing the same functions as man, that is, (a) observation, (b) processing, and (c) reaction (or, in some cases, the sequence may be reversed or modified, as found in stimulating devices). Whatever the case, to accomplish its function, the instrument must have at least three elementary "systems." These are:

1. The signal input, **detecting** or **sensing system.**
2. The signal processing or **modifying system.**
3. The signal display or **read-out system.**

Since each of these three systems is in turn made up of individual stages and component chains, some knowledge of the basic units that might be contained within a system can be useful.

THE FUNCTIONAL UNITS

The block diagram approach for a typical instrument is used in Figure 18-1. In the diagram, the transducer represents the input system; the amplifier represents the processing system; and the meter represents the display system. The functional units or circuits that might possibly be found in any one of these systems

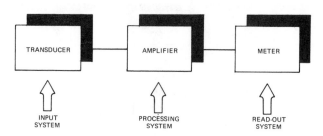

Fig. 18-1: Block diagram of the functional systems of an instrument complex

are innumerable, but there are a few that find great enough application to warrant being considered as typical examples.

In the case of input systems, the element generally used is some type of transducer; since input systems have been discussed in some detail in Chapter 17, they will be omitted in this section. We will go on to the signal processing system, which, in most cases, involves amplification and wave shaping.

Processing Circuits I—Amplifiers

The processing system can consist of a single isolated circuit or many interconnected circuits involving various feedback and timing signals and, in most cases, will involve at least one stage of amplification. Should the system involve more than one stage, it may contain a **pre-amplifier.** Pre-amplifiers are used primarily to detect very small transducer output signals; consequently, they can be summarized as *high sensitivity small signal amplifiers.*

In addition to a pre-amplifier the system may contain a **differential amplifier.** Sometimes referred to as double-ended amplifiers, these circuits are at times used to detect and amplify the difference between two input signals, but more often they are used to discriminate between the input signal and associated noise.

Also included in the system might be an **operational amplifier,** functioning in any one of a dozen different modes. With appropriate circuit design, operational amplifiers can perform various functions from voltage summation to integration or differentiation of the input signal.

In most instances the amplifier system will be required to feed

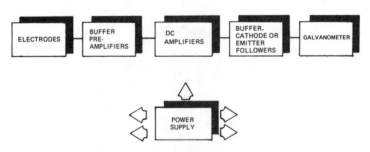

Fig. 18-2: Simplified block diagram of a typical electrocardiograph instrument complex

its output to a recorder or some other display system, which could have an impedance that is incompatible with the output amplifier stage. In this case a **buffer-amplifier** stage is used to match the circuit impedances.

A complete typical amplifier system used in ECG circuitry is shown in Figure 18-2. Note that buffer amplifiers are used at each end of the system, input and output.

Processing Circuits II—Waveshaping and Converters

For the most part, the signal voltages detected by medical instruments are either of an **analog** (constantly varying) or a **discrete** (individual pulse) nature. Most biopotentials such as nerve impulses and muscle activity are voltage pulses varying in magnitude from 50 μv to 100 mv, while analytical instruments such as colorimeters and gas chromatographs generally present output signals that resemble Gaussian curves. Figure 17-25 was a typical Gaussian curve. In both cases the information conveyed by the signal is contained in either the pulse or curve height, the pulse duration, or the area under the signal. To extract these data requires special circuitry, capable of "cleaning up" the signal by eliminating distortion and associated noise, as well as circuitry that is able to discriminate between signals of various magnitudes or frequencies.

Schmitt trigger circuits (Chapter 15) can be used to "clean up" pulses. Figure 18-3 shows a pulse input to a Schmitt trigger and the corresponding output.

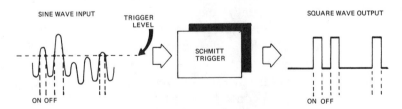

Fig. 18-3: A Schmitt trigger circuit

The terms *pulse discriminator, pulse height analyzer,* and *threshold detector* can all be used to describe a Schmitt trigger functioning to detect pulses of different amplitudes by rejecting those below a preset value, and passing only those above that value. This input threshold level is controlled by the trigger point (or bias) value applied to the circuit (c.f. Figure 15-11(B).

When information or data to be evaluated are in analog form, or are contained in the *area beneath a curve,* circuits capable of digitizing the signal are often employed.

Analog-to-digital conversion can be accomplished by either voltage comparison techniques or electronic integration, depending upon the specific requirements.

One voltage comparison method uses a **ramp function generator** (Chapter 15) to produce a voltage that shows a linear increase with time (c.f. Figure 15-8). By specially designed gate circuitry, the ramp voltage is started at the time the input is applied, both signals being fed to the comparator. The ramp voltage also triggers a constant rate counter (usually an oscillator or free-running multivibrator (Chapter 15). The counter gives an output as long as the ramp voltage is below that of the signal voltage. When the ramp voltage equals the signal voltage, the counter stops and the sequence starts over again.

Some circuits use a step voltage instead of a ramp voltage as the comparison input, but the overall circuit operation is fundamentally the same, the area under the curve being determined and converted to a digital value.

In many instances analog-to-digital conversion is performed to obtain the integral of some analog voltage. The most common methods of integration found in instruments today are *electromechanical disc techniques* and *electronic integration* (using a form of voltage-to-frequency conversion).

Electromechanical disc integrators (Figure 18-4) consist of a constant speed, motor-driven disc, upon which is placed a ball that is free to rotate. The rotational speed of the ball is directly proportional to its distance from the center of the disc. The position of the ball is controlled by the analog input voltage (or recorder pen). The ball drives a roller which is connected to a cam and the cam in turn operates a counter or a trace recorder. To explain the unit's overall function, when the input voltage is low, the ball is near to the disc's center; consequently, it rotates slowly and therefore yields a low count. As the input voltage increases,

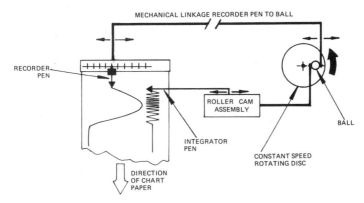

Fig. 18-4: Simplified diagram of a disc (mechanical)

the ball moves outward and its rotational speed increases, yielding a more rapid count.

Electronic integration can be accomplished by use of a **reactance tube voltage-to-frequency converter,** or a solid state **operational amplifier.**

The reactance tube voltage-to-frequency converter was borrowed from the field of FM broadcasting in which reactance tube modulators, by varying the carrier frequency around a fixed value, are used to insert intelligence into a carrier signal. The amount of frequency variation is proportional to the input voltage magnitude. In short, the bigger the input, the more cycles generated.

The same principle is applied to a method of integration and the circuit functions as illustrated in Figure 18-5. A reactance tube is connected into an oscillator tank circuit in such a way that it is

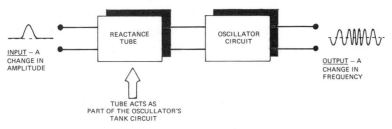

Fig. 18-5: A reactance tube integrator

equivalent to an inductance or capacitance. Its reactance varies with the value of the input signal and in turn the varying reactance changes the output frequency of the oscillator. An increase in input to the reactance tube may cause its capacitive reactance to decrease, thereby increasing oscillator output frequency, or the reverse action may take place. Whatever the case, the output frequency is always related in a known way to the magnitude of the input signal.

The use of a capacitor as the feed-back element in an inverting operational amplifier results in an integrating circuit (Figure 18-6). With minor external circuit changes (the addition of various passive elements) operational amplifiers can be made to sum integrals, integrate the same signal twice (double integrator), and even give the difference between two integrals. These devices are, without question, extremely versatile.

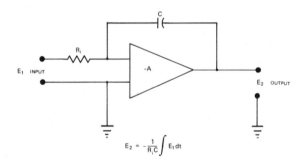

$$E_2 = -\frac{1}{R_i C} \int E_1 \, dt$$

Fig. 18-6: An integrating operational amplifier

The list of signal processing circuits is almost unlimited; the number and types of circuits used in a specific instrument is dictated only by what the signal is required to accomplish. The following paragraphs include only a few examples of some other processing circuits which an instrument user may encounter.

Phase shift circuits can be used to produce a lead or lag in a signal with reference to another; these circuits are also called **phase inverters** when they produce a full 180° phase shift (Figure 18-7).

Clipper circuits can selectively remove positive or negative peaks from waveforms, while **clamper circuits** are used to provide new reference levels for AC signals. For example, the output from an

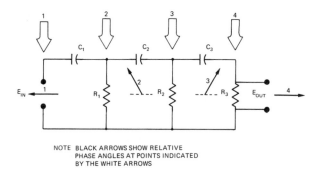

Fig. 18-7: An RC phase shifting network

amplifier may be an AC signal that varies 10 volts above and below a 0 volt DC reference. A clamper can change the signal so that it varies 20 volts above or below a 50 volt positive or negative DC reference (Figure 18-8).

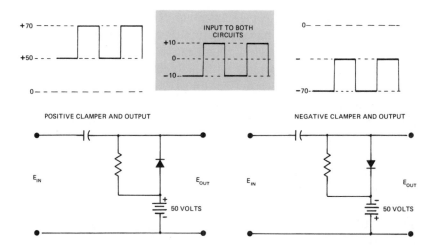

Fig. 18-8: Diode clampers

Constant frequency oscillators or multivibrators can be used as **timing** or **"clock" references** in instruments that require synchronized circuit functions. **Constant voltage** and **current** sources can be obtained by various circuit designs (primarily by use of Zener diodes) to provide reference values in many instruments for increased stability.

DISPLAY SYSTEMS

Information display or read-out methods incorporated into medical instruments run the gamut from conventional meters and galvanometers to solid state alpha numeric digital registers and ultrasophisticated, three-dimensional CRT computer displays. Information display methods are becoming increasingly complex but, whatever their form, their ultimate aim is consistent: to supply the operator with the maximum amount of information in the simplest way possible.

The most common instrument display devices are: (1) **meters** (including galvanometers); (2) **recorders**; (3) **digital systems**; and (4) **oscilloscopes**.

Meters

Meter movements generally found in medical instruments are of the string galvanometer or D'Arsonval (Chapter 4), or Weston, type, employing electromagnetic principles. A current (the detected signal) flowing through a coiled movable element produces a magnetic field which interacts with a fixed field. This interaction of the two fields produces a deflection of the movable element that is proportional to the magnitude of the detected current. The moving element has an indicator needle attached which moves across a graduated scale. (In the case of the more sensitive string galvanometer, the principle of operation is the same but, instead of an indicator needle, a mirror that reflects a light beam across a graduated scale is used.)

Iron vane, electrostatic, and dynamometer meter movements are also used in some applications, but not to the same extent as the D'Arsonval movement.

Some instruments employ a single meter movement, but have changeable scales (faces) in order that the device may be read in more than one set of units. Examples of this are found in some colorimetric instruments with which absorbance and per cent transmission or various concentration units can be read on the same instrument by changing the meter face.

Recorders

Running a close second to meters in applications involving medical instruments are **recorders**. These read-out devices are widely used in instruments from ECG and EEG applications to analytical chemistry techniques such as gas chromatography and colorimetry. Recorders are valuable because they give a permanent record of the detected signal.

All recorders fall into one of the two categories: (1) **moving coil** or **galvanometer recorders**; and (2) **potentiometric recorders**.

Moving coil (or **galvanometer**) **recorders** operate on the same basic electromagnetic principle as meter movements. The detection coil, suspended in a fixed magnetic field, is deflected by an amount proportional to the detected current due to interaction between the magnetic field around the coil and the fixed field.

These moving coil recorders can be (a) *direct writing* or (b) *indirect writing,* depending upon the type of indicator that is attached to the moving element. Direct writing types employ an ink pen that leaves a trace on untreated chart paper. The pen operates by capillary action. Other types may have a heated stylus that produces an image on heat-sensitive paper. The frequency response of a direct writing recorder is limited by the inertia of the moving element; to overcome this problem, indirect writing methods that utilize reflected light beams or ink jets were developed.

Oscillographic recorders have a small mirror mounted on the moving element of a galvanometer (much like the D'Arsonval mirror galvanometer described in Chapter 4). A light beam is focused via the mirror onto photosensitive chart paper, thereby producing a trace as the paper moves. The frequency response of this type of recorder is approximately 100 times greater than that of direct writing instruments. Other types of oscillographic recorders may use ultraviolet light beams in place of visible light. The latest instruments employing this type of readout use a self-developing chart paper.

Yet another writing method utilizes an ink jet, projecting a fine spray of ink from the capillary onto the chart paper. The capillary is either attached directly to the moving coil, or it is deflected

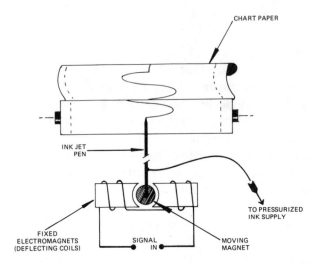

Fig. 18-9: A magnetically deflected ink-jet pen recorder

magnetically by an amplified version of the detected signal exciting two soft iron core coils between which the pen is mounted (Figure 18-9). Ink jet recorders can be obtained that have a frequency response up to 1 KHz, about midway between that of direct writing and optical recorders.

Potentiometric recorders involve a form of null balance circuitry (Figure 18-10), incorporating differential amplification and

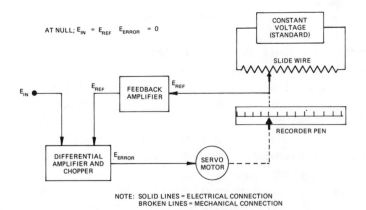

Fig. 18-10: A potentiometric null-balance recorder system

feedback control. The system is a continuous-balance circuit that compares the input signal (E_{IN}) with a reference feedback signal (E_{REF}). When the two potentials are the same, no signal is sent to the servomotor. When E_{IN} and E_{REF} differ, the differential amplifier detects the difference (called the *error voltage*) and this in turn is sent through a chopper amplifier to the servomotor. The motor drives the recorder pen and the coupled reference voltage arm until E_{REF} equals E_{IN}. The error voltage is then zero and the system is once more in balance. The reference voltage is usually tapped from the recorder slide wire across which a constant or standard voltage is applied.

Other types of potentiometric recorders (Figure 18-11) are the (a) *X-Y* and (b) linear logarithmic recorders. The first type has two sets of slide wires and servo systems, one of which (usually the *X*-axis system) supplies a time-base signal. The second type contains a separate log-amplifier and slide wire which are used for recording in the logarithmic mode and another set for linear recording.

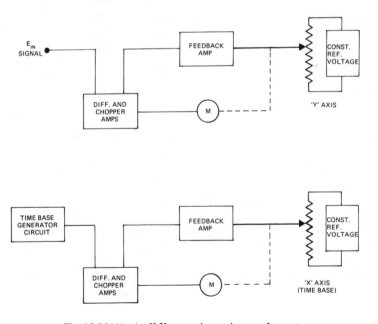

Fig. 18-11(A): An X-Y potentiometric recorder system

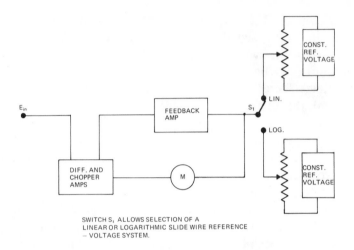

SWITCH S, ALLOWS SELECTION OF A
LINEAR OR LOGARITHMIC SLIDE WIRE REFERENCE
– VOLTAGE SYSTEM.

Fig. 18-11(B): A lin-log recorder system

Important recorder characteristics of interest to users are the instrument's *frequency range,* its *frequency response,* and its *sensitivity.* Sensitivity is usually measured in terms of deflection per unit of input (undamped), (*ie,* cm/mA or cm/μA, etc.) while response times are usually determined by measurement of the time required for the pen to span full scale in seconds or milliseconds.

Display Methods—Digital

Digital read-out or **display** methods are becoming increasingly popular in medical instrumentation, not only because they eliminate possible reading error due to parallax (*cf Glossary*) common with conventional meters, but because they are also generally more accurate.

The two most common forms of digital display techniques are (1) **electromechanical registers** and (2) **electronic** (tube or solid state) **indicators.** While both types of display are capable of yielding numeric information, only the electronic systems are widely used for alpha-numeric information displays (letters as well as numbers being displayed). Most mechanical displays found in medical instruments are of the *coupled wheel* or *drum* type, with numbers from 0-9 printed on each wheel. These displays may be driven by a stepping motor or an electromechanical (ratchet-type) step relay.

In both electromechanical and electronic systems, some form of analog-to-digital conversion of the signal is required in order to produce counting pulses.

Mechanical displays have an upper frequency limit of 15-20 Hz; consequently, they cannot be used in applications that require rapid, high-number counting (as in radioisotope or particle counters) without some stages of **frequency division** being incorporated prior to the signal reaching the meter.

Mechanical displays find widest use in instruments designed for colorimetry, spectrophotometry, flame photometry, and other opto-analytical chemistry techniques. One reason for this is the fact that the response of mechanical displays is compatible with the types of signals generated in these techniques. Three other advantages of electromechanical registers are their *low cost, unsophisticated driving circuitry,* and *insensitivity to shock and vibration.*

The most common and oldest of tube type alpha-numeric indicator is the **nixie**, or cold cathode tube. When filaments (formed as letters or numbers) are stacked in a tube containing neon gas, application of the required voltage to the appropriate filament causes it to glow, indicating a letter or number. The device is limited in that generally no more than 12 characters can be contained within one tube. A second limitation is the relatively   high driving voltage (150 v approximately). Nixies are advantageous in that they require relatively simple drive circuitry when compared to other tube and solid state indicators.

A second tube type indicator contains seven individual filament segments that can be selectively energized to form alpha-numeric characters (Figure 18-12). Segmented type tubes require a lower driving voltage than the conventional nixie tube but more complex drivers.

The area of greatest activity in display devices today is in solid state design, in which two of the newest indicator sources are the **L.E.D.** and the **planar glow panel.**

The L.E.D. is a gallium arsenide *light emitting diode* that is smaller and less power consuming than other indicator types. It

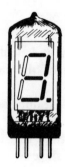

Fig. 18-12: A typical seven segment display tube, with the character 'three, decimal' illuminated

operates at 1.75 volts with a current of 50 mA. These indicators are usually seven-segment displays with a life expectancy comparable to conventional solid state devices.

Another type of L.E.D. alpha-numeric display is made of 36 single dot diodes in an *X-Y* array that allows an extremely high versatility in character formation (Figure 18-13).

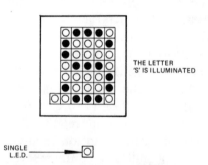

Fig. 18-13: An X-Y array indicator using L.E.D.'s (light emitting diodes) (courtesy Monsanto Special Products, Cuperton, Calif.)

A different operating principle drives **planar panel solid state displays**. These units are a type of dot matrix configuration utilizing 111 single cathode-double anode (front and back), gas-discharge diodes. When a dot is to be shown on the indicator the front anode is utilized; at all other times the glow is transferred to the rear anode and is not visible on the panel front.

Figure 18-14 shows a simplified cut-away view of this form of display.

By far the most widely used display device for visualizing electrical activity is the **cathode ray oscilloscope** (CRT). This device has found application as an electronics tool with a value unmatched. The heart of an oscilloscope is its cathode ray tube and its versatility extends from graphic computer three-dimensional displays to monitoring biopotentials and outputs from analytical instruments. Recently CRT's have begun to find application in the area of alpha-numeric display techniques, but they are not extensively used due to the complex circuit requirements of display positioning, blanking, and symbol or character generation, etc.

All of these tube and solid state indicators generally require decoder and driver circuits in order to function. These circuits are, for the most part, integrated (logic) circuits that accept the digitally coded input information and transmit outputs to the appropriate light elements. It is the decreasing cost of indicator drive circuitry that is making semiconductor digital displays more economical and consequently more prominent in today's instrument marketplace.

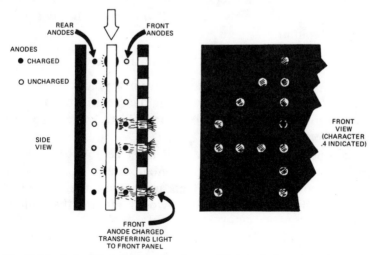

Fig. 18-14: A simplified diagram of a planar solid state display system (courtesy, Burroughs Corp., Plainfield, N.J.)

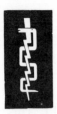

a closer look at some common circuits

CHAPTER 19

Once an electronic circuit has been designed, its value and its applications are limited only by the imagination and ingenuity of its users. It seems that a few circuits have almost infinite adaptability and as a result can be found in a great number of instruments. Although a brief description of some of them was given in the previous chapter, a slightly more detailed discussion will be attempted in this chapter.

The greater part of the following material is devoted to various special amplifier circuits, primarily because the amplifier is without question the most widely applied and adaptable electronic circuit encountered by instrument users.

Since all amplifier designers seek to produce a circuit that approaches the ideal, the characteristics they desire in a circuit should first be collectively discussed under the heading of the "perfect" amplifier.

THE "PERFECT" AMPLIFIER

The perfect or ideal amplifier is, from a practical viewpoint, impossible to build. However, by listing the specifications the ideal amplifier should possess, one is more able to evaluate practical working amplifiers.

To be a perfect amplifier, a circuit must be able to accomplish its function as if it were virtually nonexistent; that is, it must amplify without having any effects upon the circuits associated with it. To do this, an amplifier would require the following characteristics:

1. Zero input power;
2. Infinite output power;
3. Infinite input impedance;

4. Zero output impedance;
5. Perfect linearity;
6. Infinite band width (range);
7. Instantaneous response;
8. Infinite gain.

Obviously such characteristics are (at least for the present) not within the grasp of the electronics industry. However, consideration of these desirable characteristics enables us to define the specifications for a good, practical amplifier. Since the first two "perfect" characteristics violate the law of conservation of energy, we will dispense with them and begin with the third: input impedance.

A good amplifier must have a *high input impedance* to prevent loading the signal source. This is especially true of amplifiers used to detect signals such as those found in biomedical applications. However, after having detected a signal, the amplifier itself becomes a source for the next circuit (indicator, meter, recorder, etc.) in which case it should also exhibit a *low output impedance.* In the process of amplifying a signal, the gain of the circuit should show a constant value throughout the whole spectrum of possible input signals; in short, the gain must be *linear* over its whole band width. In order to accommodate rapidly changing input signals (*ie,* high frequency signals, pulses, etc.) an amplifier must have fast *response,* commonly referred to as frequency response. Finally, in order to modify the input signal into a practically usable value, the amplifier must have *high gain.*

Few practical amplifiers have all these characteristics, but as the sciences of electronic design and engineering materials advance, the devices produced become closer to being the perfect amplifier. It should be noted that although the circuits described in the following sections are classed as amplifiers, they differ from the previously discussed basic circuits in that they generally contain two or more tube (or transistor) stages, at times packaged within a single container.

DC AND CHOPPER AMPLIFIERS

The biopotentials and transducer output voltages that constitute the vast collection of signals fed into medical instrumentation fall into two general classes: (1) DC and low frequency analog signals, and (2) AC signals.

DC amplifiers are characterized by the fact that the signal to be amplified is directly coupled to the input of the amplifier. Such signals are generally slowly changing DC potentials, and they act as small variations in bias, thereby causing subsequent variations in the output of the amplifier. Due to the problem (found in virtually all electrical systems) of **drift**, DC amplifiers with high gain were, until recently, difficult (and expensive) to produce. As all electronic components are sensitive to environmental conditions of temperature, electric and magnetic field, etc., slight potential changes can cause variations in amplifier output without any input signal present; this constitutes what is known as *amplifier drift*. Only since the advent of the operational amplifier have practical and economical high gain DC amplifiers become possible. Before that time, in order to combat drift, it was more economical to design additional circuitry and use a concept from broadcasting called *modulation* to build chopper amplifiers.

The term **chopper amplifier** is somewhat misleading in that the amplifier itself is not a chopper but rather a conventional audio frequency amplifier. It is the additional circuitry of mechanical or electrical chopper, modulator, and demodulator sections that make up the complete chopper amplifier system or stage. Figure 19-1 shows a block diagram of a chopper amplifier system, the operational sequence of events, and the pertinent wave forms.

The basic operating concept behind a chopper amplifier is as follows:

1. A constant frequency, constant amplitude sine or square wave signal alternately turns on and off an amplifier or interrupts its input. (This is the carrier signal.)
2. With no input (modulation) signal to the amplifier, the output is a sine or square wave.
3. This sine or square wave is then passed through a demodulator that mixes a second identical carrier with the first, in such a way that the two signals cancel, and no output results.
4. If modulation, a change in the magnitude of the carrier caused by an input signal, does occur, when it is mixed with the demodulating signal, the *difference* between the two is

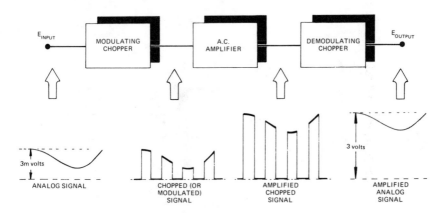

Fig. 19-1: A chopper amplifier system

detected and passed by the demodulator, yielding as an output an amplified version of the input signal.

The modulator or the chopper section in these amplifiers can be one of four types:

1. A mechanical chopper, employing a vibrating reed type mechanism that is electromagnetically controlled (Figure 19-2A).

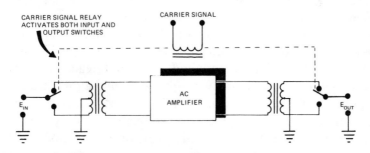

Fig. 19-2(A): A relay operated chopper amplifier system

2. A diode "pad" with an oscillator (carrier signal) input.
3. A double vacuum tube or transistor chopper with carrier input.

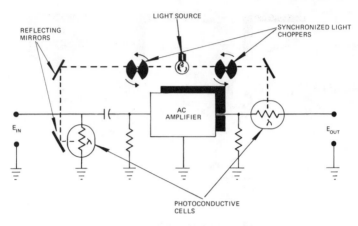

Fig. 19-2(B): A photoelectric chopper system

4. A photoelectric chopper employing a motor-driven vane to interrupt light paths (Figure 19-2*B*).

In most instances the same type of chopper control section is used in both front-end (modulator) and output (demodulator) circuitry, and the same carrier signal source feeds both sections.

DIFFERENTIAL AMPLIFIERS

A class of AC amplifiers that constitute a large segment of special amplifier circuits used in analytical instruments are the **differential** (or **null balance**) type amplifiers.

Conventional amplifiers are of the single-ended (single-input) variety; a term used to indicate that the input signal is injected between a single input lead and a ground lead. In contrast, **differential amplifiers** have two input leads and a third lead which is common. When signals are applied to both input leads, the amplifier output is a magnified reproduction of only the *difference* between the two. Any signal voltage common to *both* leads is not passed by the amplifier. This action is extremely helpful in rejecting electrical noise. Electrically generated noise such as 60Hz power line noise, thermal noise, or shot noise, will appear on both the reference and measuring lead, while the detected signal appears on only the measuring lead; consequently, the amplifier action passes only the detected signal, effectively rejecting the electrical noise. The ability of such circuits to block unwanted potentials in this manner is called **common mode rejection** and may be expressed as a figure of merit, being the ratio of differential input over common input.

Some dual beam (or signal path) analytical instruments, such as flame photometers and colorimeters, utilize a type of null-balanced differential amplifier in their read-out circuitry. Initially the amplifier is balanced to read zero with the instrument's reference side and test side signals applied and no detected input present. When the detected phenomenon causes variation in the test side signal voltage, the differential output is proportional to the detected signal. Figure 19-3 shows this principle as it can be applied to a dual beam colorimeter. Note that the output is the difference between transistor collector potentials. The voltage in turn causes deflection of a galvanometer. The potentiometer in the collector circuit allows the operator to null-balance the system initially whenever the inputs are slightly unequal due to minor component or circuit variations.

It is interesting to note that such null balance circuits can actually be considered as Wheatstone bridges that amplify, the transistors functioning in place of the variable resistors in a conventional resistance bridge.

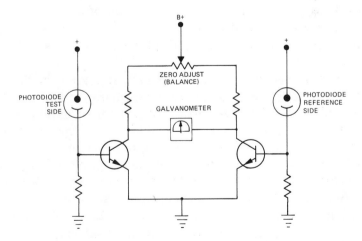

Fig. 19-3: A differential or null-balance amplifier in a dual beam colorimeter

BUFFER AMPLIFIERS

A special type of amplifier circuit common to bio-instrument systems is the **buffer amplifier**. Buffer amplifiers are used to link circuits that would otherwise be mismatched with regard to relative input and output impedances. Field effect transistors and cathode (or emitter) followers are utilized in buffer amplifier circuits, since they have the desirable characteristics of relatively high input impedance and low output impedance. The gain of impedance matching circuits is not a primary concern (it is close to unity), since the amplifiers in the following stages will generally accomplish whatever amplification of the signal is required.

PRE-AMPLIFIERS

Pre-amplifiers (high sensitivity amplifiers) are used in applications in which very small signals (at times in the microvolt range) are to be detected. These circuits not only require high gain and sensitivity, but in addition must exhibit a high input impedance to prevent loading the signal source. Absence of a high input impedance results in signal distortion. The circuits are usually push-pull amplifiers capable of producing considerable gain.

OPERATIONAL AMPLIFIERS

Operational amplifiers are the most versatile and flexible class of amplifiers available, spanning such applications as computer signal processors, mathematical function operations, signal comparators, multivibrators, DC amplifiers, and a host of other circuits.

These invaluable circuits were originally developed in the field of computer technology to perform mathematical operations. The primary characteristic that distinguishes their operation is their predictable gain, the magnitude of which is a direct function of the form of negative feedback employed in the circuit.

Basically, these devices are direct-coupled high-gain amplifiers. The addition of a negative feedback network with resistive or capacitive elements modifies their operation such that the gain of the system becomes a precise function of the feedback signal produced. In Figure 19-4, the triangle symbolizes the basic operational amplifiers, while R_I and R_F are the input and feedback resistances. The output of this circuit can be found by multiplying the input voltage E by the ratio of R_F/R_I so that:

$$E_O = E_I \cdot \frac{-R_F}{R_I}$$

(The negative sign implies the 180° phase inversion found in a conventional amplifier.)

With proper selection of R_F and R_I, very high gains with an accuracy often as good as 0.1 percent are possible.

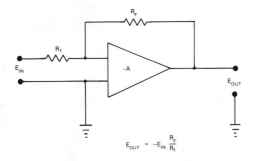

Fig. 19-4: A typical operational amplifier schematic

Replacing R_F with a capacitor of the appropriate size will yield an integrating circuit (Figure 19-5), while replacing R_I with the same capacitor produces a differentiating circuit (Figure 19-6). Other configurations of the basic operational amplifier circuit can be made to produce voltage summation, differential input opera-

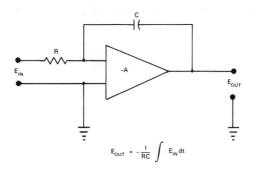

Fig. 19-5: An integrating operational amplifier

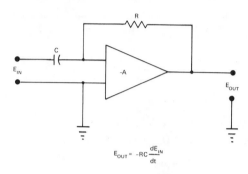

$$E_{OUT} = -RC \frac{dE_{IN}}{dt}$$

Fig. 19-6: A differentiating operational amplifier

tion, signal comparison, and voltage or current reference sources. These devices are utilized in innumerable biomedical instruments, from electrocardiographs and electroencephalographs to data-processing equipment. Although they do not possess the characteristics of the "perfect amplifier," they come relatively close and their wide flexibility is an outstanding advantage. One important disadvantage of operational amplifiers is *offset,* which refers to the small output voltage (consisting of AC noise and a DC component) produced when no input signal is present. Usually the amplifier's offset specification is given by the manufacturer as the amount of input voltage required to yield a zero output. By the correct use of biasing circuits, this problem can be controlled. In most instances, for operational amplifier accuracy, the manufacturer will also include any drift error to be used in gain calculations, drift error being the change in offset due to temperature variation, aging, etc., and expressed in microvolts per degree, or day, respectively.

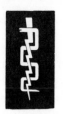

power supplies

CHAPTER 20

Every electronic instrument requires some source of energy to function. In clinical instrumentation, the most common sources of operating power fall into one of three categories: (a) **transformers**, (2) **batteries (dry and wet cells)**, and (3) electronic power supplies.

TRANSFORMERS

Transformers are especially designed and constructed coils used for the purpose of transferring energy from one circuit to another without a wired connection between the two. Basically, a typical transformer consists of two wire coils wound around a common metallic core and electrically insulated from each other (Figure 20-1). Color-coded leads provide connections to the coils and the whole assembly is mounted within a metal case. Energy from one circuit (the primary) is transferred to the other circuit (the

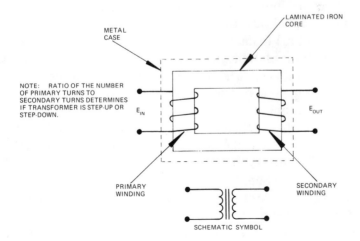

Fig. 20-1: A simplified diagram of an iron core transformer

225

secondary) as follows: Current in the primary coil produces a magnetic field which is concentrated by the iron core. The magnetic field interacts with the secondary coil, inducing power into it. Power in the secondary coil is usually between 90 and 98 percent of that originating in the primary, making transformers an efficient and practical means of transferring electrical energy.

By selection of the correct ratio of the turns in the primary coil to those in the secondary, transformers capable of stepping up or down the primary voltage can be produced. If a transformer steps up voltage, the current in the secondary will be less than that in the primary, and vice-versa. This should be obvious since the power produced in the secondary ($P = E \times I$) cannot be greater than that introduced in the primary.

Transformers find many applications in electronic instruments, their most common uses being (1) *to supply power* to an instrument, (2) *to isolate circuits* or stages, and (3) *to couple circuits* or stages having mismatched impedances.

Depending upon its application, the secondary coil of a transformer can consist of a single winding or it can have multiple windings, as in the case of typical instrument power supplies in which the transformer supplies high voltage for rectification as well as low voltage and filament outputs. Whatever the case may be, all windings are usually identified by standard color-coded leads: the line input leads are generally **black**, the high voltage secondary output leads are **red** with a **red and yellow** striped center tap lead, and tube filament leads are **green**.

Another type of transformer common to many clinical instruments (*eg,* Autoanalyzer, Coleman Spectrophotometer) is the **constant voltage transformer**. By selective construction and alignment of the primary and secondary coils and the inclusion of a captive element, constant voltage transformers supply a steady output voltage from the secondary, even though the voltage applied to the primary may vary over a relatively wide range. They are used often to supply a constant voltage to electro-optical instrument light sources to ensure a steady level of illumination.

Isolation transformers are used in many clinical instruments as a safeguard to prevent anyone receiving an electrical shock from touching both the instrument and a grounded metal object as well as to supply the power necessary to operate the equipment.

Autotransformers are special types of power sources that employ only one winding which is tapped. They have the advantage of yielding a relatively constant output to a varying load, but also the disadvantage of not isolating, electrically, the primary circuit from the secondary. Autotransformers are capable of yielding variable secondary voltages; a well-known brand is *Variac*. By changing the position of a movable secondary tap along the secondary winding, different values of output voltage are obtainable.

BATTERIES

Batteries of one form or another constitute a wide class of power sources in equipment in which relatively small (compared to transformer-driven devices) amounts of energy or instrument mobility is required. They are also often used in applications demanding very steady values of DC voltage, not normally obtainable from electronic supplies without considerable expense. One common application of mercury dry cell batteries is as the reference cell in an instrument potentiometer circuit such as that found in the Coleman Universal℗ spectrophotometer and the Buchler-Cotlove chloridimeter℗.

Battery power sources are made up of cells which come in many shapes and sizes, from the round, all purpose, everyday flashlight dry cell to the **mercury** and **alkaline** cells having very stable outputs. A comparison of the three most common dry cells is given in Table 20-1.

TABLE 20-1

COMPARISON OF TYPES OF DRY CELLS

Characteristic	Zinc-Carbon (Flashlight type)	Zinc-Mercuric Oxide (Mercury cell)	Zinc-Manganese (Alkaline cell)
Stability	Least stable	Most stable	Intermediate
Storage life	6-12 months	Up to 2 years	Up to 2 years
Life in use	Relatively low	4-5 times zinc-carbon	3-5 times zinc-carbon
Cost	Low	High	High

The **zinc-carbon** type dry cell output voltage degenerates gradually as the battery is used, while in contrast the mercury cell voltage remains constant right up to a few minutes before it fails (Figure 20-2).

Wet-cell or secondary type (storage) batteries are more generally found in automobile and industrial applications and not usually in clinical instrument applications (an exception being the old Beckman DB Spectrophotometer).

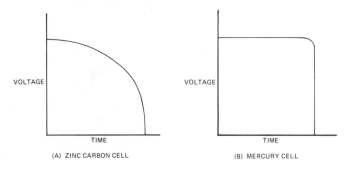

(A) ZINC CARBON CELL   (B) MERCURY CELL

Fig. 20-2: Simplified comparison of the voltage degeneration curves for ZnC (A) versus Hg (B) cells

ELECTRONIC POWER SUPPLIES

In all instruments requiring high levels of DC energy, electronic supplies are normally used to obtain the operating power. A typical electronic power supply can be divided into five stages as shown in Figure 20-3. The function of each of the stages is as follows:

1. **Transformer:** The input transformer supplies a stepped-up voltage in the secondary (*ie,* 120 v primary to 450 v secondary) and isolation from commercial power lines. In some tube-type instruments it also supplies stepped-down voltage for tube filaments.

2. **Rectifier:** The rectifier changes the AC voltage to a pulsating DC, either half wave or full wave, dictated by design and application.

3. **Filter:** The filter network employs capacitors (which oppose a change voltage) and sometimes choke coils (inductors,

which oppose a change in current) to smooth out the pulsating DC into an average or effective DC voltage.

4. **Regulator:** The voltage regulator maintains a steady DC output that might otherwise change with fluctuations in the load current. (See Chapter 2 for a review of loading and its effects.)

5. **Divider:** The voltage divider network provides different DC voltages for the various circuits within the instruments.

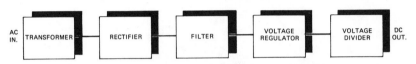

Fig. 20-3: A block diagram of a typical electronic power supply

The quality of a power supply can usually be determined by an examination of its detailed specifications and component parts. A good general rule of thumb to follow is "the heavier, the better." Good quality power supplies have heavy transformers and full wave rectifiers as well as both capacitive and inductive filtering. Not all power supplies have voltage or current regulation; this is dictated in most instances by the quality and application of the instrument as a whole.

Metallic and Silicon Rectifiers

Although high voltage vacuum diodes are used in many instances to provide the rectification within a power supply, two other types of rectifiers are used at times to provide the same action.

Metallic or **dry disc rectifiers** (Figure 20-4) are constructed of stacks of dissimilar metal plates (copper-copper oxide or silicon-iron). Current flows more easily in one direction than the other across the metallic interfaces, and consequently the device is able to rectify an alternating current.

Silicon diodes operate in the same fashion as the semiconductor junction diodes described in Chapter 13. These semiconductor rectifiers can supply DC currents ranging from two or three to five hundred amperes. In some clinical instruments they are found mounted at the back or underneath the chassis so that any heat

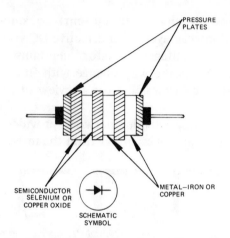

Fig. 20-4: Pictorial diagram of a metallic rectifier

generated by their operation can be dissipated directly to the metal chassis.

A form of rectifier often used to produce higher DC output voltages than the transformer secondary voltage is the **bridge rectifier**. Either vacuum tube, metallic, or silicon devices may be used in the construction of this type of circuit. Twice as much voltage output can be obtained from a bridge rectifier, as compared to a conventional full wave rectifier having the same transformer secondary voltage. The available current, however, is only half as good.

Filter Circuits

The most common method of removing the variations or "ripple" from a pulsating DC voltage is with an **electrolytic capacitor**. The capacitor, placed in parallel with the rectifier and

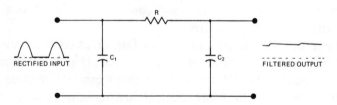

Fig. 20-5: A capacitive input filter circuit

load (Figure 20-5), charges to the maximum potential of the pulsating DC. When the rectifier voltage begins to drop off, the capacitor discharges through the load maintaining a supply of power. The capacitor can be thought of as a storage point or reservoir, supplying energy only when the rectifier fails to do so. It is recharged again by each succeeding DC "pulse."

Chokes or iron core coils are inductors usually found in power supplies yielding high currents. Since inductors function to oppose a change in current, chokes are connected in series with the load (Figure 20-6), often in conjunction with a filter capacitor.

In instrument applications calling for very low values of ripple (almost pure DC) multiple stages of filters can be used. They may be of the capacitive input *pi*-type or the choke input *T* type, the prefix designation referring to the way in which the components are connected. Figure 20-6 is a capacitive input *pi*-type filter.

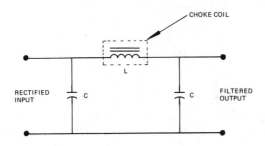

Fig. 20-6: *A capacitive input L-C filter employing a choke coil (L)*

Voltage Regulation

Voltage regulators are found in the power supplies of instruments having critical DC requirements for operating purposes and in which the load variations cannot be handled by a conventional unregulated supply.

The three methods of obtaining voltage regulation are (1) **glow tube** or **gas-filled** voltage regulators, (2) **electronic** voltage regulators and (3) **Zener diode** regulators (described in Chapter 16).

Whenever the amount of current drawn from a power supply changes, the change is reflected back as an increase or decrease of

currents within the supply itself. Without some form of stabiliza-
tion, such internal current changes would result in variations of
the output voltage.

A common method for accommodating such fluctuations in
load current while maintaining a constant voltage utilizes gas-
filled, cold cathode glow tubes.

In a *glow tube regulator,* once its gas is ionized, any variation in
load current changes only the *degree* of ionization. The amount of
ionization in turn controls the resistance of the tube. If ionization
increases, (increased current) then resistance decreases proportionately so that the voltage remains constant. Since $E = IR,$ if a rise in
current is accompanied by a proportional reduction in resistance,
the product E remains unchanged (Figure 20-7). The current
changes that can be handled by a glow tube regulator determine
the range of its operation. To cope with load fluctuations beyond
the capability of a single tube, various series and parallel
arrangements of tubes are used.

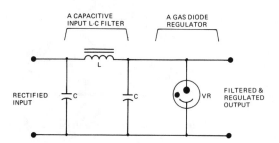

Fig. 20-7: A voltage regulator circuit employing a gas diode (glow tube) regulator

Electronic voltage regulation involves a type of feedback
control mechanism. In the circuit shown in Figure 20-8, the
output voltage appears across the resistance consisting of R_1 and
R_2 in series. Any changes in load current tends to cause changes in
E_{OUT} and in the current through R_1 and R_2, thus causing a
change in the grid voltage on tube V_2. Plate voltage on V_2 then
shows an opposite change. This action in turn, since it is felt at the
V_1 grid, causes either increased or decreased conduction through
V_1. The action of V_1 compensates for any tendency to change in

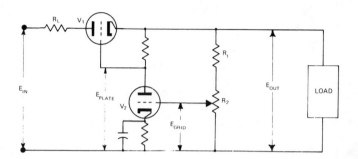

Fig. 20-8: Basic elements of an electronic voltage regulator (see text for explanation)

the voltage across R_1 and R_2, thereby keeping the output voltage stable. *Zener diodes* or gas diodes are often used in V_1 cathode circuits to provide a constant reference bias voltage.

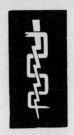

SECTION III

medical electronics
and bioengineering

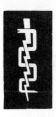 # the art of trouble-shooting

CHAPTER 21

When a physician is faced with the problem of diagnosing the cause of a patient's ailment, his task is not unlike that of an instrument user who may be plagued with a faulty flame photometer, an erratic EKG recorder, or some other device which is giving unreliable readings. But, whereas many health workers are very willing to match wits with the physician in attempting to speculate as to the cause of the patient's problem, utilizing their common sense and knowledge of physiology, anatomy, microbiology, etc., few (if any) are willing to use that same approach and information provided by instrument manufacturers to diagnose a "sick" instrument, mainly because very few have ever had pointed out to them the similarities that exist in tackling both problems. This analogy may sound far-fetched, but just a quick look at the "design" features of both the human body and instruments from a common point of view will make the relationship clearer.

The human body is an infinitely complex unit consisting of numerous physiological subsystems interconnected by fluid, electrical, and chemical pathways. However, this arrangement is not unlike the design incorporated into an electronic instrument, for an instrument may consist of five or six separate electronic subsystems, just as functionally connected by metallic conductors. Circulating hormones and chemicals found in the blood act as a form of feedback control in mediating the functions of the body; voltage-mediated feedback control mechanisms are just as common in instrumentation (servo recorders are a good example). There is not an instrument built today that can compare with the complexity of the human body. Why then are many instrument users more ready to attempt to solve problems in human systems than in much less complex electronic "bodies"? The answer to that question is the basis for this chapter; simply put, they don't know where to begin. The information contained in the following pages will hopefully provide the worker with a foothold from which to advance into this seemingly never-never land of "trouble-shooting."

THE REQUIREMENTS

Although the analogy between the human body and an electronic system is a highly simplified one, nevertheless, trouble-shooting a faulty electric instrument is just as much an art as is trouble-shooting a sick body. As with any art, it is developed through *knowledge* coupled with *experience*. Just as a physician is required to know his physiology, biochemistry and anatomy, etc., and to couple this with experience, an individual attempting to trouble-shoot electronic instruments must have a knowledge of electronics, the operating theory of the instrument, and experience in using test equipment. The "electronic physician" attempting to diagnose an instrument fault has a much less complex unit to deal with than a physician faced with a sick patient. However, there is only one master circuit design of the human body, even though the packaging of the assembly varies (for which we males are most thankful) but electronic instrument designs and circuits vary according to their applied function and can be quite confusing. By use of a few common denominators, however, this problem *is* surmountable.

The following summarized requirements, though incomplete, are, in the author's opinion, a few of the more important essentials with which a worker attempting to trouble-shoot a piece of electronic instrumentation should be familiar. However, this does not apply to "shock therapy technicians" (those who believe a swift kick or thump in the right place will solve any problem). The requirements are:

1. Some knowledge of basic electronics.
2. Ability to use electronic test equipment (generally limited to a volt, ohm-milliammeter, but may also include an oscilloscope).
3. Ability to read schematic and block diagrams (not as difficult as it seems as will be shown later).

4. Knowledge of some common denominators found in electronic instruments.
5. Common sense (which, sadly, seems to be an increasingly uncommon attribute).

Items *1* and *2* of these requirements are obtained by formal or self-study (and since the reader has reached this point in the book, it is not unfair to assume he has some knowledge of both) while item *5* is in us all (we hope). The remainder of this chapter deals with items *3* and *4* which are the key elements in any attempt at trouble-shooting.

BLOCK DIAGRAMS—THE BEGINNING

As was pointed out in Chapter 18, electronic instruments are made up of subsystems. These subsystems consist of circuits, which are in turn made up of component chains.

The word *circuit* is a somewhat indefinite term since it can often be used to describe either a single network or, in some instances, discrete systems that contain two, three, or more simple circuits, as found in an oscilloscope (Figure 21-1). An oscilloscope's sweep circuit, which this author prefers to consider a subsystem, contains two, three, or more basic circuits such as oscillators, amplifiers, etc. To simplify matters and present a uniform method of approach to analysis, *any network consisting of two or more basic circuits or stages (amplifiers, filters, etc.) will be designated a* **subsystem.**

In addition to an understanding of the system (or block diagram) approach, a few facts basic to all instrument diagrams, although they are obvious, are seldom recognized by many people involved with using the diagrams. These **common denominators** are:

1. The circuitry in every electronic instrument consists of numerous *DC* (or *power flow*) *paths* and one or more *signal* (or information/intelligence) *paths.*
2. Every individual circuit has a *DC path* which functions to establish the circuit's DC potentials the instant power is applied to the instrument.
3. Every individual circuit has a *signal path* along which fluctuations in potential are used to produce signal (or information) transfer.

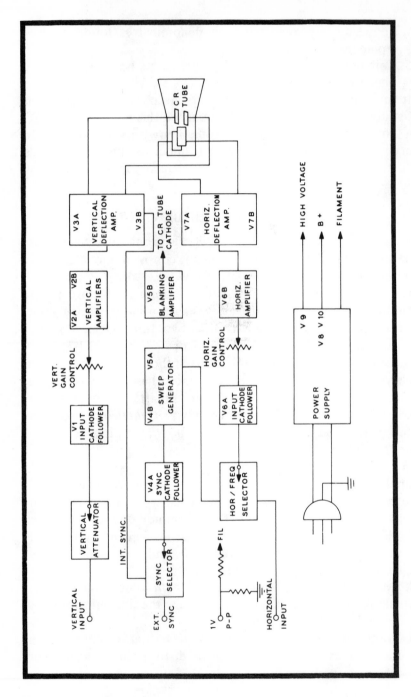

Fig. 21-1: Block diagram of an oscilloscope made by the Heath Co.: Model IOW-18 (courtesy Heath Co.; Benton Harbor, Michigan)

4. These two paths (DC and signal) are usually represented *perpendicular* to each other in block and schematic diagrams.
5. *DC paths* are run from *ground* to the *power supply*.
6. *Signal paths* usually run *input* to *output* (oscillator circuit to output in the case of a stimulator or similar signal-generating device).

Figure 21-2 shows a typical schematic diagram with the DC paths indicated by dark solid lines, and the signal paths indicated by light broken lines.

Instrument manufacturers generally supply the purchaser of a product with three things: (1) an *instruction manual,* (2) a *block diagram* of the instrument, and (3) in some cases, a *schematic diagram.* The **block diagram** functionally breaks the instrument down into its subsystems and circuits, generally designating within each block the tubes or transistors that are a part of that particular circuit. In addition, it may also indicate the signal path by arrows— circuit to circuit. A most important point that should be re-emphasized is that *by convention, signal paths run left to right across schematics and block diagrams.* The term *signal path,* as used in this sense, refers either to an external signal injected into an instrument (*eg,* an ECG pulse injected into an oscilloscope) or a signal generated or arising within an instrument that is required for its operation (*eg,* the internal sweep signal in an oscilloscope).

Figure 21-1 shows the block diagram of an oscilloscope in which there are two major signal paths, both terminating at the same point: the cathode ray tube. One is the horizontal sweep signal; the other, the input or vertical signal. The four major subsystems into which this particular instrument conveniently divides (Chapter 18) are, excluding the CRT: (1) power supply, (2) vertical input (circuit), (3) horizontal input (circuit), and (4) sweep generator (and associated circuits). Note that the block diagram showing these systems identifies the tubes associated with each circuit. This small amount of information can be extremely valuable in trouble-shooting. For example, assume that the oscilloscope in Figure 21-1 shows horizontal deflection of its electron beam, but no vertical deflection. This reaction is an indication of trouble in the vertical amplifier section. A simple check of the block diagram permits the appropriate tubes/

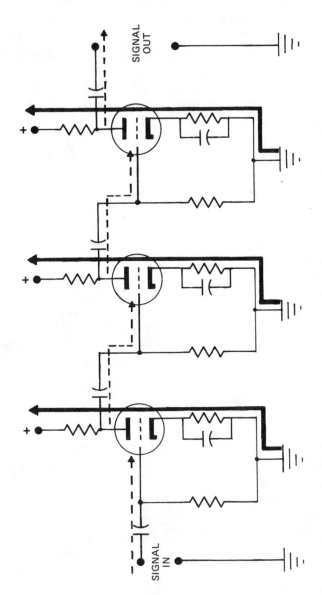

Fig. 21-2: A three stage amplifier circuit. Signal path indicated by a broken line, major DC paths by solid lines

transistors in the vertical input amplifier subsystem to be identified by number and then removed and examined. Without the use of the block diagram, and unless one is familiar with their layout and identification, all the tubes would have to be tested. A simple block diagram trouble analysis such as this can, in many cases, save a great deal of wasted time.

In many instruments being manufactured today, block diagram analysis is the most that is required when trouble-shooting, since the major part of their circuitry consists of plug-in circuit "cards" or "boards." These printed circuits contain all the active and passive components involved in the circuit's function, mounted on a mica or plastic support board and connected by paths of conductive material instead of wires (Figure 21-3). All connections to power sources and associated signal processing circuits are made by way of special snap-together plugs. When a problem has been isolated to a particular board, it is removed and another one is snapped into place; then we are ready to go!

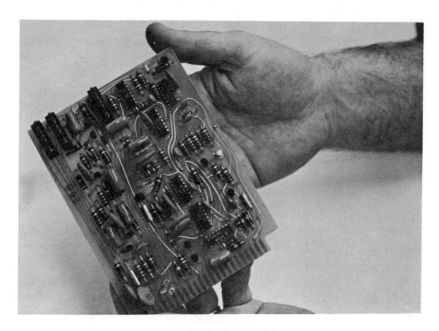

Fig. 21-3: Photograph of a printed circuit board

THE SCHEMATIC DIAGRAM AND SIGNAL TRACING

The information in this section is intended primarily for those individuals who have had some experience in trouble-shooting but who have not been exposed before to a systematic approach or *modus operandi.*

After a block diagram analysis has determined the tubes or transistors that *may* be causing the trouble and, assuming these in turn have been checked and found to be good, the probable indication is trouble at a component level: a broken wire, burned-out resistor, or blown capacitor, etc. To trouble-shoot at this level requires utilization of a **schematic diagram**—or, as they have been called by some instrument users, "spaghetti diagrams" or "nightmares." Although at first glance the densely packed symbols and lines seen in a schematic tend to make the unfamiliar user nervous, knowing a few basic facts about them and having an ability to recognize component symbols soon make schematic diagrams appear much less "unfathomable."

The first point a potential trouble-shooter should keep in mind is that component failure in an instrument circuit inevitably results in a break or deviation of a *signal* or *DC path* which will manifest itself in some way, either by nonoperation or incorrect operation of the instrument. The symptoms of the problem can be obvious or they can be obscure, but they *will* be there.

A second important point for trouble-shooters to keep in mind is that, unless one is thoroughly familiar with an instrument, analysis by schematic should never be attemped without prior reference to the block diagram. *First,* use the block diagram to signal trace and determine what *circuits* may be involved with the loss or distortion of the signal. *Second,* find the location of the involved circuits by locating the numbers on the tube(s) or transistor(s) in the block diagram, and then identifying them on the schematic. Let us look at an example. The signal generator shown in Figure 21-4A has a problem that manifests itself as *no squarewave output.* Reference to the block diagram tells us that between the points of signal generation and output, there are four tubes and one passive circuit involved: (A) V_1 and V_2, the **bridged-T oscillator**; (B) $V_4 A$, the **input cathode follower**; (C) $V_5 A$ and B, the **Schmitt trigger circuit**; (D) $V_4 B$, the **output cathode**

follower; and (E) the **passive circuit output attenuator.**

Now refer to the schematic diagram in Figure 21-4*B*. Note that each subsystem can be located and identified by using the tube numbers given in the block diagram.

The system of interest is on the right: the squarewave circuitry (*Note:* in this instance, *not* in the same relative location as shown in the block diagram). Immediately one can see that V_1 and V_2 (the oscillator tubes) are a *6CB6* and *12BY7*, respectively. The input cathode follower ($V_4 A$) is one-half of a *6AW8,* and the Schmitt trigger consists of both halves of a *12AT7* ($V_5 A$ and *B*). The output cathode follower ($V_4 B$) is the other half of the *6AW8.*

Now that the individual circuits have been located the next step is to trace the DC paths for each of them. (A good rule of thumb to follow is: begin at ground, finish at the power supply.) For an example let's try $V_5 A$:

1. Begin at ground, through *R-35* to pin *3* on the cathode. Continue through the tube, cathode to plate, pin *1*; on through *R-33* and the R.F. choke coil to *R-37*, and then to the *271 VDC* supply (which, you will find by referring to the power supply section, connects to the top of *C-22*).

2. For tube $V_4 A$ (the input cathode follower), the path is as follows: ground, *R-27, R-26,* pin *(1)* $V_4 A$ - pin *(3)* $V_4 A,$ *R-28, R-37,* to *271 VDC.* Now see if you can trace the paths for V_2 *and* V_3. (The correct solutions are given below the diagrams.)

Tracing signal paths is a little more difficult than following DC paths, but not impossible if an additional concept is kept in mind: in tube type circuits, the signal is generally *injected on the grid* and *taken out at the plate.* This is true unless the circuit is a *cathode follower* in which case the signal is taken out at the *cathode.* In transistor circuits the problem is a little more complex since we must first know if the circuit we are dealing with is a common-base, common-emitter, or common-collector.

Look again at Figure 21-4. To locate the problem existing in the square-wave circuitry requires the trouble-shooter to identify the signal path components involved, and then check along to determine where the signal is lost. The signal is initiated as a sine wave at the bridged-T oscillator. Depending upon the position of

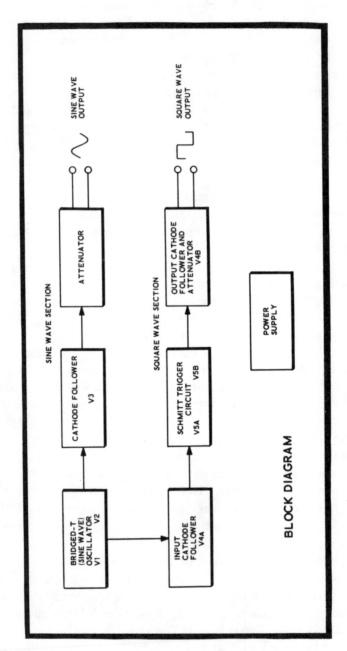

Fig. 21-4(A): Block diagram of a Heath sine-square wave generator. Model EUW-27 (courtesy Heath Co., Benton Harbor, Michigan)

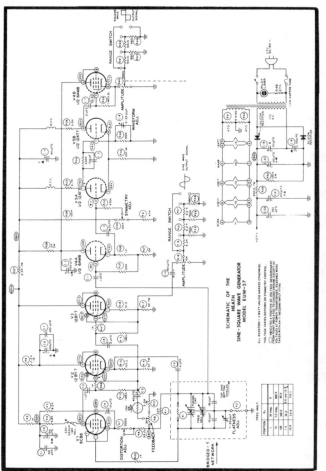

Fig. 21-4(B): Schematic diagram of the Heath sine-square wave generator. Model EUW-27 (courtesy Heath Co., Benton Harbor, Michigan)

DC path solutions for Tubes V_2 and V_3 (Figure 21-4):

 V_2: *Ground, R-14, R-13, pin (1) V_2, pin (7) V_2, R-6, 271 VDC.*

 V_3: *Ground, R-17, R-16, pin (1) V_3, pin (7) V_3, 271 VDC.*

the range switch, the signal will pass through the following circuits; from the bridged-T network, by way of C-11 to pin (2), grid
of $V_4 A$. At this point a question must be answered: where does
the signal come out of $V_4 A$? It can be answered in the following
way. By referring to the block diagram, one can see that $V_4 A$ is
listed as a *cathode follower*. The answer is in the name; the signal
is taken off the cathode! Another way of determining the signal
exit point is by tracing *back* from the grid of $V_5 A$ (pin (2)) to see
where it is originating in the previous stage. Continuing, the signal
leaves $V_4 A$ cathode, pin (1) and arrives at the grid of $V_5 A$ pin (2)
by way of C-13. It exits $V_5 A$ at the plate, pin (1) passing through
an RC network consisting of R-34 and C-15, to the grid of $V_5 B$
pin (7). Leaving the plate of $V_5 B$ pin (6), the signal passes through
C-17 to pin (7), the grid of $V_4 B$, and exits through the output
cathode follower from pin (6), through R-40 (amplitude adjust)
on through the range switch to arrive at the output jacks.

Most schematic diagram analysis can be approached in a similar
manner, and consequently can make what seems to be an
insurmountable problem a little easier. The worker must also
remember that *effective* trouble-shooting requires the following:

1. A proper method of approach (hopefully supplied by the
   information in this chapter).
2. Some knowledge of the theory of operation of the instrument (and basic electronics).
3. A logical thought process (cause-to-effect reasoning).
4. An ability to read diagrams and use test equipment.
5. Concentration.
6. Patience.

Lucky guesses may help once in a while, but a little deductive
reasoning will save many hours of frustration and wasted time and
money. However, remember that instrument problems have an
irritating way of showing themselves in illogical ways and at odd
times. Although locating the problem areas requires, among other
things, logic, they themselves do not provide such logical clues and
at some times they must be approached very much like a tangled
ball of string.

A TROUBLE-SHOOTING CHECK LIST

The general outline of the step-by-step procedures to use in trouble-shooting an electronic instrument should follow a method similar to that given in Table 21-1.

TABLE 21-1

TROUBLE-SHOOTING CHECK LIST

A. Check to see if AC power is applied (at the wall outlet).

B. Check to see if the instrument is plugged in and turned on.

C. Make a visual inspection for blown fuse, burned-out components, loose wires, shorted wires or components, etc. (Use your nose! Overheated components such as resistors and insulation have a very distinctive and disagreeable odor.)

D. Make a visual inspection to see that all tubes have filament voltage (look for the glow in the tube). A tube that normally glows red will glow bluish when it becomes leaky.

E. Using a block diagram of the system, try to isolate the problem to a particular stage.

F. Using the schematic diagram, measure DC voltage. (Voltages at points such as plate, grid, cathode, or supply are usually indicated by the manufacturer on the schematic.)

G. With power off, make continuity checks (open or short) of DC paths. (In the process, remember how capacitors and inductors react to ohmmeter checks—Chapters 5 and 6.)

H. Injecting a signal at the input circuit (front end), use an oscilloscope to trace the signal path. If it appears at the input of one circuit but not at its output, you have isolated the faulty circuit.

By adhering to these rules of trouble-shooting procedure and applying the knowledge you have of your instrument, you should be able to develop self-confidence and proficiency and be able to isolate *most* instrument problems.

As a point of interest you may want to know what the author considers are the most probable causes of instrument "failure." In order of highest probability they are:

1. The instrument is not plugged in, or turned on.

2. A blown fuse.

3. The instrument is O.K.; the operator does not know what he is doing. (Don't laugh—it's not as far-fetched as it seems.)

4. Dead or weak tubes, transistors, etc. The greatest number of

vacuum tube failures result from either low emission, open filaments, or internal shorts—transistors just open.

5. Misalignment and/or calibration.

6. Circuit problems (bad components).

An instrument is only as good as its operator; keep this in mind.

In many instances, if a particular tube, transistor, or circuit board is suspect, replacing it with a good one from stock or another good instrument will usually tell whether or not it is faulty.

Table 21-2 should give some idea of a few common problems that can be associated with an instrument's faulty operation. The list is by no means complete and it is meant only to provide the worker with a base from which he is able to expand his knowledge and develop his own mode of diagnosis in the area of instrument trouble-shooting.

COMMON INSTRUMENT PROBLEMS

TABLE 21-2

GENERAL TROUBLE-SHOOTING CHART

Indication	Probable Source of Trouble	Check (By or At)
1. No power	a. Power cord not plugged in	Visual inspection
	b. Switch is off	Visual inspection
	c. Fuse blown	Visual inspection
	d. Faulty switch	Voltmeter check
	e. Bad power supply tubes	Tube test
2. No signal (at display or output)	a. No input or generated signal (not properly connected)	Signal source
	b. Faulty input/output circuit/ transducer (stimulator or electrodes, etc.)	Input/output connector or transducer
	c. Faulty modifier circuits or display device	Check involves extensive trouble-shooting to determine bad tubes/ meter circuit boards, etc.

TABLE 21-2 (Continued)

GENERAL TROUBLE-SHOOTING CHART

Indication	Probable Source of Trouble	Check By (or At)
3. Erratic signal (Sometimes it is there, sometimes not)	a. Loose connection(s) solder joints—internal tube shorts, etc.	Tap all wires, tubes with the eraser end of a pencil while watching signal indicator
	b. Interference due to radiation, electrostatic, electromagnetic, and leakage	Move away from location of power transformer motors, generators. Check shielding and grounds!
	c. Faulty tubes, transistors to power supply-modifier circuits	Check tubes, transistors, circuit boards (by substitution of a spare), etc. etc.
	d. Faulty components, leaky capacitors, etc.	Visual check (look carefully; a leaky electrolytic capacitor usually has a small pin hole in its end or a gel-like material oozing out of it)
4. Unstable base line (zero-drift)	a. Faulty power supply tube/ transistor*	Replacement required
	b. Faulty modifier tubes	Replacement required
5. Nonlinear signal	a. Instrument is out of calibration	Calibrate
	b. Nonlinear amplifiers	Check tubes/transistors
	c. Nonlinear tuned circuits	Retune circuits (electronic technician's job)
6. Noisy signal (Signal is there, but unstable)	a. Radiated noise	See 3b
	b. Internal noise	Check shielding and grounds; check for leaky components, gassy tubes

*In the case of photometric instruments the phototubes/photomultiplier should first be checked as well as the light source.

A STITCH IN TIME! – PREVENTIVE MAINTENANCE

Although this chapter has dealt mostly with an approach to trouble-shooting, in a large number of malfunctioning instruments the problems that arise and require trouble-shooting can usually be prevented if a system of preventive maintenance is established for each instrument and adhered to. With the amount of use that most diagnostic and analytical instruments are subject to in today's medical centers, preventative maintenance is a must. It is obviously better to have an instrument "down" at a time when you can organize and schedule your way around its absence than to have it fail right in the middle of a high load period or when it is attached to a patient.

A few items to keep in mind that might serve as a basis for developing a periodic maintenance check list (also keeping in mind the instrument manufacturer's recommendations) are:

1. It does not hurt to check all tubes in an instrument once every six months. Some tubes give immediate indications of failing, while others deteriorate slowly.
2. Cleanliness is efficient: this includes mechanical, optical, chemical, and electrical systems. Impurities such as dirt, dust, oil, etc. (dust plus moisture = a conductor):
   a. In mechanical systems, can cause excessive wear.
   b. In optical systems, can cause erroneous results due to light path interferences. (Problems may arise due to spillage or leakage as well as lamp blackening from oxidation of spilled chemicals.)
   c. In chemical systems, can cause electrical leakage paths and high resistance connections (the result of leakage and spills of corrosive chemicals).
3. Properly ground your instruments (*cf,* Chapter 24). Stray ground potentials, as well as being hazardous, can prevent consistent accuracy.

Three parting reminders!

1. If you don't know what you are doing, *don't do it.*
2. Before putting *hands in motion,* be sure *brain is in gear.*
3. *Think!* Then, *good luck* and *good hunting.*

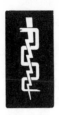 clinical ECG monitoring and
electroencephalography

CHAPTER 22

The field of physiological measurement has progressed a long way since the days of the "foot-in-a-tub" electrocardiograph. An overwhelming number of measuring and monitoring instruments can be found in today's modern hospitals, and these medical aids are being developed so rapidly that new equipment sometimes becomes obsolete before it blows its first fuse. Today's medical practitioner—whether physician, nurse, or technologist—must be familiar with a large amount of medical instrumentation falling under the classification of monitoring and stimulating equipment. A great many volumes could be written (and a few have been written) describing the instruments used to monitor blood pressure, heat rate, pulse rate, respiration, and various other parameters. This chapter is meant to serve only as a descriptive introduction to the most common clinical monitoring techniques for those who are uninitiated in this rapidly expanding field.

The physiological parameters most often observed in hospital operating rooms, and intensive and coronary care units (where most clinical monitoring equipment is found) are the electrocardiograph (ECG) data, blood pressure, heart rate, respiration rate, blood pH, and blood gases (pO_2, pCO_2). Evaluating the status of a critically ill patient involves continually studying various groups of these data. A typical system that considers each one of these areas will be outlined to briefly describe the components and the general design features involved.

ECG MONITORING

The human body has more than once been described as a "bag of electrolyte solution with its own electrical system." The life processes within this "bag" are initiated, controlled, and evaluated by thousands of electrical pulses, voltage changes, and chemical reactions, and the classical central element in this organic complex is the heart. The heart is a magnificent natural pump whose pumping action is stimulated by electrical activity generated at the *sino-arterial node* with rates varying from 55 to 95 beats/minute in the average adult. Due to the excellent conducting ability of the body, the activity of the heart can be monitored at the body's surface with the use of the right technique and equipment.

The signal produced by cardiac activity and detected at the skin's surface is approximately 1 millivolt in amplitude, varying in frequency from 0.1 to 100 Hz (Hz = Hertz or times per second).

It is assumed that most readers are familiar with the electrophysiology of the heart; therefore, only a brief summary will be given in order to relate the heart's electrical activity to the characteristic ECG waveform as shown in Figure 22-1:

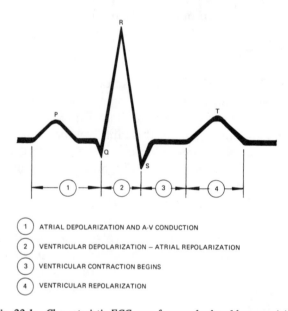

Fig. 22-1: *Characteristic ECG waveform and related heart activity*

1. **The P wave and P-R interval:** produced by depolarization of the atria and conduction through the atrioventricular node.
2. **The QRS complex:** produced by ventricular depolarization.

3. **The ST segment and T wave**: produced by ventricular repolarization.

The equipment used to monitor cardiac activity can be simplified, and divided into four subsystems:

1. Transducers (electrodes);
2. Pre-amplifiers;
3. Amplifiers (differential/operational/other);
4. Display equipment.

The electrodes used in electrocardiography are not transducers in the strict sense of the word (Chapter 17), since no energy conversion takes place within them. More accurately, they can be considered as conductors linking the body surface to the measurement system.

Electrodes used in electrocardiography vary in design and size; some of the more commonly used types are: (1) plate electrodes, (2) suction (cups) electrodes, (3) floating disc electrodes, (4) needle electrodes, and (5) spray-on electrodes, developed by the National Aeronautics and Space Administration (NASA). A new development in electrode design has been experimented with in the Scandanavian countries. Conductive silicone rubber ECG electrodes have been developed that supposedly eliminate many of the problems associated with conventional metallic electrodes.

Intracardiac needle electrodes are sometimes employed for monitoring purposes in research applications but usually not in routine applications. Figure 22-2 shows some of the more popular electrodes in use today.

All of the electrodes used in electrocardiography come in one of two functional designs; they are either (1) *direct-contact* or (2) *floating electrodes.*

Direct-contact electrodes require the metal element to be in direct contact (hence the name) with the skin. **Floating electrodes** ride on a layer of electrolytic jelly or paste interspaced between the skin and metal. For short-term applications, such as office use, direct-contact electrodes are adequate, but in instances requiring long periods of use, such as ICU and CCU patient monitoring, floating electrodes are superior. (Some hospitals do use needle electrodes for this purpose, however.) The widespread preference for floating electrodes is a result of extensive evaluation of the

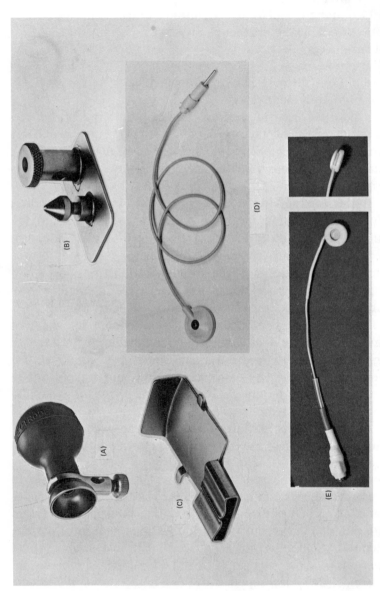

Fig. 22-2: *ECG electrodes (A) suction cup (B) limb electrode (C) plate-limb electrode (D) fluid column - silver/silver chloride (E) fluid column - german silver (A-D courtesy Hewlett Packard Co. Waltham, Mass.) (E - courtesy Mennen-Greatbatch Electronics, Inc., Clarence, N.Y.)*

various factors that can affect electrode performance; they have proven to be most versatile. These performance factors can either (1) modify the detected signal, (2) cause drift potentials, or (3) produce extraneous signals (voltage artifacts). The first two problems are common to all electrodes in almost any application, and therefore can be called *fixed* performance factors. The latter problem may or may not occur, depending upon the particular situation and consequently can be termed a *variable* performance factor.

Some *fixed performance factors* are:

1. The *type* of metal used. Human skin has a characteristic response to each metal used in an electrode. Active metals, (for example, copper) produce ionization which can cause polarization and poor electrode response.
2. The *temperature* and *humidity* of the electrode environment can change the impedance of the skin-metal interface.
3. The detected signal's *frequency* must be matched by the response of the electrodes. Most physiological electrodes tend to show a high impedance (opposition) to low frequency signals and less impedance to higher frequencies.
4. The *size* of an electrode determines the current density across the skin-electrode interface and, consequently, the resulting signal reproduction.
5. In the case of floating electrodes, the *paste* or electrolyte used produces its own characteristic skin response.

The *variable factors* affecting an electrode's overall performance and producing interfering potentials are:

1. Variations in *electrode composition.*
2. *Changing* interface *impedance* resulting from movement of the electrode.
3. Muscle potentials due to patient *motion* or involuntary muscular activity in surrounding tissues.

Of the previously mentioned ECG electrodes, the types usually encountered in monitoring are all variations of the disc type, silver/silver-chloride floating electrode. The major differences among the many types of commercially obtainable disposable electrodes are: (1) the type of adhesive used to secure them and (2) the method of lead-to-electrode attachment.

The largest percentage of operating problems encountered in monitoring can be traced to a single cause: **poorly applied electrodes.** Although the correct method is ridiculously simple to master, many individuals approach electrode application with an attitude that borders on negligence. The tendency to slap on a wad of electrode paste and plop an electrode onto it seems to increase in proportion to the number of times the activity is performed. This is asking for trouble. Three items must be considered when applying ECG electrodes in order to insure good contact and trouble free signal reproduction. *First:* the electrode paste. Electrode pastes are conductive fluids, especially formulated to decrease skin to electrode impedance. Substituting other solutions (*ie,* isotonic saline) does *not* accomplish the same purpose. *Second:* the skin itself. Since normal human skin offers a high resistance to current, it must be adequately prepared. It should first be properly cleaned (with alcohol), then a little electrode paste applied and thoroughly rubbed in. A slight reddening will occur if this is done correctly. Incorrect electrode application as well as dirty or corroded electrodes result in poor electrode-to-skin continuity, generally manifested by a wide wandering baseline in the displayed waveform, called "60 cycle" noise. In an attempt to overcome this problem, experienced users advocate periodic changing of electrodes, in some cases by each nursing shift, or, in other cases, each day. Although this practice further raises the probability of artifact generation, in most instances, with due care in the application of electrodes, including correct preparation of the skin, there is really no reason why they cannot be left in place for at least twenty-four hours (except possibly in the case of an allergic response on the part of the patient).

Proper electrode application calls for careful attention not only to the choice of electrode paste and preparation of the skin but also, of importance when using chest leads, to the use of an adequate amount of electrode paste—but not too much (it's not *how much* you use, it's *how well* you apply it). Due to the close proximity of chest leads, inaccurate recordings can be obtained if the paste overlaps. To be absolutely sure of good continuity, commercial electrode-to-skin continuity checkers are now available that eliminate the guesswork.

Even with correct and trouble-free electrode application, the best metal electrodes are prone to some artifact generation, caused by skin stretching, muscular activity, etc. In an attempt to circumvent such problems, some European researchers have experimented with *conductive silicon-rubber electrodes.* The silicon electrode adapts to the skin contour, is somewhat adhesive, and is chemically inert. Tapping these electrodes while in use produces no distortion in the trace. These electrodes supposedly offer the advantages of low impedance (used with conventional electrode paste), low artifact production, and prolonged use without irritation.

Most modern monitoring equipment has, incorporated into its circuitry, an electrode-fault-detecting system. A typical unit consists of a high frequency oscillator whose signal is transmitted from one electrode (usually the common, or leg, electrode) and detected by the other two. The frequency of the fault signal is high enough so as not to interfere with the ECG itself. After the electrodes have been firmly attached to the patient, the fault-detecting system is activated and set to transmit its signal across the electrode-patient impedance. Should any electrode work loose, the inter-electrode impedance is altered, decreasing the magnitude of the signal being sensed and consequently triggering the alarm circuit. To ensure that movement artifacts do not trigger the system, a time delay (*eg,* 15 seconds) is designed into the circuit preventing the actual alarm from triggering until the time interval has passed.

ECG Pre-Amplifiers

The various low magnitude signals encountered in physiological monitoring (ECG, EEG, EMG, etc.) must all be amplified anywhere from one thousand to one hundred thousand times before they are of a practical magnitude for evaluation. To accomplish this, without at the same time amplifying noise artifacts and other extraneous signals, requires the use of selective, sensitive, high gain pre-amplifiers (at times referred to as *buffer amplifiers*).

The requirements for a good physiological pre-amplifier are:

1. *High input impedance,* in order not to draw current from the

biopotential source and thereby distort the signal reproduction.

2. *Good frequency response,* in order to produce accurate signal amplitude determination. To accomplish this the amplifier must respond to high frequency (rapidly changing) signals with the same accuracy with which it reproduces low frequency (slowly changing) signals.

3. *Good noise rejection characteristics,* in order to eliminate 60 Hz AC common-mode (present on all leads) and differential AC (relative lead-to-lead values) potentials, as well as skin surface DC voltages, all of which interfere with accurate ECG signal reproduction. In short, the amplifier must reject all potentials except the one being investigated.

4. *Low output impedance,* in order to yield maximum signal transfer to the next stage.

5. *Selectable bandwidth,* in order that the system can be used either for long-term conventional monitoring (when narrow bandwidth is used) or short periods of diagnostic study (when wide bandwidths are used). The range of frequencies (bandwidth) to which the instrument responds is then easily selected for either purpose by way of a switch.

Figure 22-3 is a pictorial representative of the impedances and potentials developed at the skin electrode interface due to *contact polarization* at the electrodes and *externally radiated* 60 Hz energy.

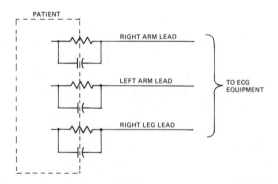

Fig. 22-3(A): Pictorial representation of skin to electrode impedances (ECG)

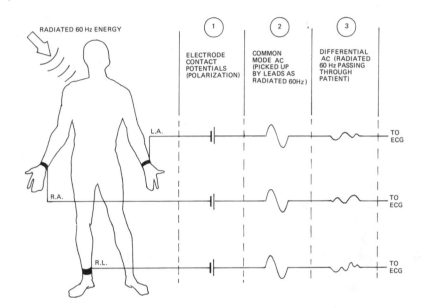

Fig. 22-3(B): Noise potentials in ECG monitoring

The pre-amplifier in a monitoring system is, after the electrodes (or transducers), the next most important stage since it is within the pre-amplifier that the signal is initially processed for removal of noise and amplified. No matter how good the rest of the system is, a poor pre-amplifier means a poor signal at the display unit or recorder.

In bedside monitoring systems, the pre-amplifier and subsequent processing stages are contained within the same cabinet or chassis. In the case of remote monitoring systems, in which signals from a number of patients are fed into a central nurses' console, the pre-amplifier can be located at the bedside or close to the patient, insuring that a good quality signal arrives at the central console.

ECG Function and Driver Amplifiers

Once the pre-amplifier has amplified, filtered, and generally prepared a good-quality, noise-free reproduction of the ECG signal, the waveform can be coupled to various types of function circuitry. Function circuits may consist of a series of DC amplifiers operating in the differential mode and feeding the signal to a voltage or power amplifier which in turn drives a recorder, galvanometer, or oscilloscope display. Other research-type function circuits can be multiple stages of operational and integrating amplifiers designed to extract information from the signal, such as the *PR, ST,* and *RR* intervals, or the area under the *P, QRS,* and *T* segments, all of which can yield diagnostic information.

Next to amplifiers, the most common type of function circuit encountered in monitoring systems is the *tachometer* or *rate computer,* which is used to detect and indicate the heart rate. This measurement is accomplished by the tachometer circuit sensing the *R-R* interval of the ECG wave and from it computing the rate. The circuit operates as a frequency-to-voltage converter, yielding an output signal whose magnitude is proportional to the input signal's (ECG) frequency. Although the peak of the *R* wave is predominantly selected as the trigger point for heart-rate computing, many manufacturers supply equipment with a manual adjustment allowing selecting of the trigger point anywhere along the ECG wave complex. In addition, adjustable high and low rate limits are incorporated into most equipment to detect instances of

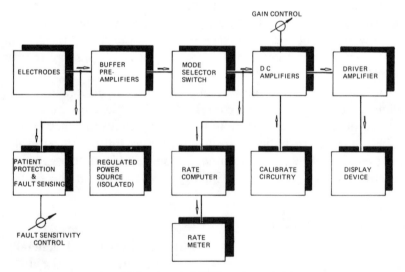

Fig. 22-4: A typical ECG monitoring system

bradycardia (decreased heart rate) or tachycardia (increased rate) with simultaneous activation of audible (clicks) and visual (flashing lights) alarms.

Various other forms of functional amplifier circuitry can be found in research equipment involved in ECG monitoring, but for the purpose of general clinical monitoring, the elements just described serve as an example. Figure 22-4 shows a block diagram of a typical ECG system.

ECG Display Methods

In hospital monitoring systems, whether bedside, central, or operating room, the oscilloscope serves as the primary form of display device. The types of oscilloscopes found in the active ICU and CCU units around the country today can supply single channel (or trace), dual channel, or even eight channel viewing so that a nurse stationed at a central console is able to evaluate the status of many patients at once. The cathode ray oscilloscopes employed in these viewers contain up to eight individual controls for adjustment of various factors such as the *brightness, gain,* and *trace speed* of each channel. Trace speeds can usually be varied from twenty-five to one hundred millimeters per second to accommodate various heart rates.

The operation of a **multiple trace oscilloscope** (Figure 22-5) differs from that of a conventional single trace device in that with single trace operation, the signal being detected is processed through the vertical amplifier section to produce vertical deflection (up and down) of a single recurring trace that without deflection would just look like a straight horizontal line on the screen. In contrast, the multiple trace oscilloscope functions as follows:

1. A conventional horizontal sweep generator provides scanning of the electron beam (deflection) across the viewing screen.
2. A high frequency vertical sweep generator provides scanning up and down the screen.
3. Blanking circuitry cuts off the electron beam completely when no input signals are present from the ECG sources. In this condition the screen is entirely clear except that flat traces are visible.

4. Each ECG channel supplies a signal to its own individual, video gating (control) amplifier.

5. An output from any of the video gating amplifiers unblanks the beam within a pre-determined space on the screen—with 4 ECG channels this means the beam is unblanked four times

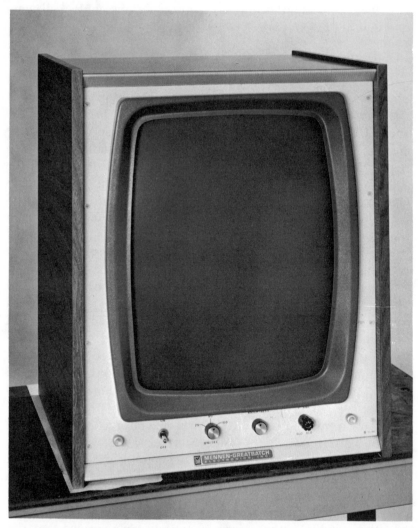

Fig. 22-5:   A four channel monitoring oscilloscope. (courtesy Mennen-Greatbatch Electronics Inc., Clarence, N.Y.)

during *one* vertical sweep—causing the signal to be reproduced on the viewing screen.

Figure 22-6 shows how an ECG pattern emerges through the synchronized sweep, blanking, and unblanking of a single electron beam.

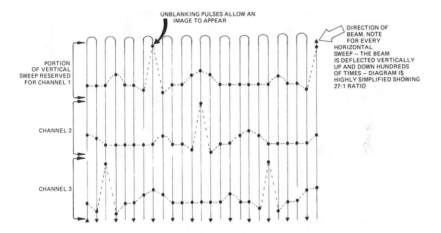

Fig. 22-6: *Simplified diagram showing three ECG channels exhibited by time-synchronized blanking and unblanking of a single electron beam*

The operation of these multiple trace oscilloscopes is very similar to the operation of an ordinary home television set in which, instead of only four gating pulses of equal intensity occurring per scan, many pulses of various intensities occur, resulting in production of a picture.

Figure 22-7 shows a simplified block diagram of typical multiple (four) trace oscilloscope system. The control and logic timing circuitry allows the input ECG signal to unblank the sweep only during predetermined time periods of the vertical sweep. In other words, a definite time segment of each *vertical sweep* is reserved for each channel.

In ECG monitoring the next most common information display technique involves the use of sensitive and highly sophisticated chart recorders. Just as oscilloscopes can be single or multiple trace (channel) recorders can also produce single or multiple

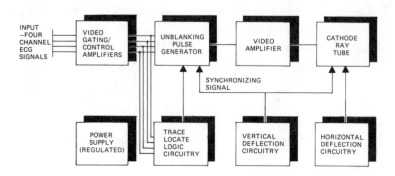

Fig. 22-7: Simplified block diagram of a commercial multiple channel monitoring oscilloscope (courtesy Mennen-Greatbatch Electronics, Inc., Clarence, N.Y.)

tracings. However, each channel in the recorder system must have the following components:

1. *A pen motor,* to drive the pen in the vertical directions (up, down).

2. *An input amplifier,* to process the weak ECG signal into a form capable of driving the pen motor.

3. *A pen* or *stylus,* which records on the moving chart paper. A single chart drive motor can be employed to serve multiple recording channels and adjustment of the chart drive speed is usually available to allow better definition of the trace in patients with tachycardia or bradycardia. Chart speeds can be varied from approximately 20 mm to 60 mm/second.

Each individual channel is usually supplied with manual adjustments for changing trace size and position as well as controls for varying stylus temperature and damping *(stylus vibration control).*

All ECG chart recorder systems operate as a form of null-balanced feedback-controlled detector that compares the input signal (ECG) against a reference signal that is developed by the pen or stylus position (Chapter 18). Any difference between the input potential and the reference potential causes the pen to move until the two are equal. Consequently, the pen is constantly tracking the changes in the input signal, yielding a permanent trace of those changes.

Other types of display techniques used in monitoring systems involve electromagnetic meters that make available information concerning heart rate, blood pressure, respiration rate, and even temperature. The meters used in these instances generally contain high quality D'Arsonval (or Weston) type movements (Chapter 4) with minor modifications incorporated into them to enable setting and *detection of high or low heart rate or blood pressure faults.* In conjunction with meter displays, coded light displays are also sometimes used. Such visual indicators might contain five lights (for instance, a central green indicator with amber indicator on either side of it and red indicators at the two outer positions). As long as the monitored parameter remains within the preset limits the green indicator is illuminated. Should the signal *approach* either the upper or lower limit, the appropriate *amber* indicator light comes on. If either the upper or lower limit is *violated*, the associated *red* indicator blinks on and off and an audible alarm sounds. The blinking red light immediately identifies both the failed channel and the patient and virtually no time is lost in attempting to identify which trace or monitor is involved. In many instances of ECG monitoring, any time an alarm is triggered, an automatic ECG tracing is taken at either the bedside or central station so that a record of the patient's condition is immediately available for the physician.

ELECTROENCEPHALOGRAPHY

Activity within the human brain results in various electrical potentials being developed due to, as postulated by some, the polarizing effects with *neurons* (nerve cells). By placing electrodes in various experimentally determined "ideal" locations around the skull or even within the brain itself, recordings of this activity can be obtained. Knowledge of the "normal" pattern of activity when compared to abnormal recordings is invaluable to a physician investigating for brain disorders due to injury or disease.

The characteristic elements of recorded electroencephalographs are:

1. *Small potentials,* ranging 10-200 microvolts with no fixed amplitude.
2. *Varying frequency waveforms,* approximate range 1-100 Hz.

3. *Identifiable frequency groups*, labeled as (a) *alpha* (α); (b) *beta* (β); (c) *theta* (θ); and (d) *delta* (δ).

The EEG wave groups are classified by frequency range; beta waves have the highest frequencies and delta waves the lowest. Table 22-1 gives the approximate frequency ranges of the four primary EEG waves.

TABLE 22-1

Alpha	α	=	8-13 Hz
Beta	β	=	13-30 Hz
Theta	θ	=	4-7 Hz
Delta	δ	=	1-3 Hz

The EEG instrument system follows fundamentally the same basic design as that used in ECG monitoring, but is somewhat larger in size due to the number of channels used (up to 24 in some instruments). The system consists of (1) *electrodes*, (2) *a signal processing unit*, and (3) *a display system* (Figure 22-8).

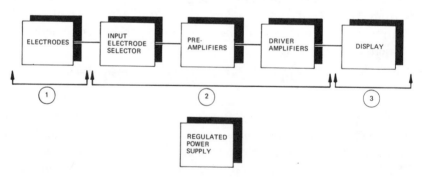

Fig. 22-8: Block diagram of an EEG instrument system

The electrodes used in EEG systems can be of three general types: (1) *solder pellets*, used with electrode paste; (2) *silver discs*, 8 to 10 mm in diameter, also used with electrode paste; and (3) *subcutaneous needle electrodes* inserted beneath the scalp. The latter type yield information with less artifact than the other two.

The various problems associated with the use of ECG electrodes apply also to EEG electrodes and must be taken into consideration during EEG recording. Signal transfer problems are considerably amplified due to the smaller size of the EEG potential. In some instances, the small pellet-type electrodes are attached with conductive cement to the patient's scalp to reduce movement artifact.

Two special methods of EEG electrode placement enable the clinician to study either localized cortical areas or general brain activity. A *monopolar* arrangement, in which one electrode is attached to a predetermined point and the other located at some point distant from the skull, serves the latter purpose, while *bipolar* connections are used to evaluate activity directly between two prepositioned electrodes.

The amplifier system used to process an EEG signal is fundamentally similar to that found in ECG instrumentation. The frequency responses of the amplifier systems are also similar since both the EEG and ECG fall within the same frequency range: 1-100 Hz. The EEG amplifiers should, however, have better low frequency characteristics. The major difference between ECG and EEG processing circuitry is the gain of the EEG system. The gain requirement of the amplifiers in an ECG system is about 1,000, while an EEG amplifier system must be able to provide an increase in signal magnitude of approximately 10,000. To accomplish this as many as four stages of amplification are sometimes required.

To display the EEG signal a four-channel recording system is used, one channel for each primary waveform, alpha, beta, theta, and delta. An individual pen and pen-centering control are also provided for each channel. EEG recorders use ink pens in contrast to the ECG heated stylus technique, and the recording chart speeds can be varied from 10 to 30 millimeters per second.

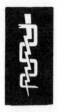 # other clinical monitoring techniques

CHAPTER 23

CENTRALIZED STATIONS

In many hospitals today, due to acute shortages of physicians and nurses, the trend in ICU and CCU unit design is toward centralized monitoring stations in which a single nurse can monitor two or more patients. The reason for this trend stems not only from an acute shortage of coronary care nurses (at least at the time of this writing, 1972) but also from other factors such as the emotional stability of patients when faced with observing their own physiological parameters on bedside equipment. Sudden activation of a bedside alarm system, due to any one of a dozen possible equipment malfunctions (loose electrodes, circuit malfunction, or loss of battery power, etc.) not associated with, or caused by, a change in his condition, can place the patient in a highly agitated condition. Under such circumstances the possibility of frightening a patient to death is not far removed; he may very well think the equipment is predicting and he is observing his own demise!

Most manufacturers of monitoring systems follow the practice of modular design with the equipment they produce. These types of "black box plug-in" units allow great versatility in choice of system design. Each monitored parameter is processed via an individual module that can be incorporated or omitted from the system at the discretion of those involved in the system preparation. A typical four-bed CCU unit may be designed as in Figure 23-1:

1. Three beds equipped for normal CCU monitoring. Parameters to be measured are:
   (a) ECG by display scope.
   (b) Heart rate computer with automatic alarm system and meter read-out.
2. The fourth bed may be equipped for a patient having an

extreme heart abnormality with equipment including the first two measurement modules plus a pacemaker unit, a defibrillator, and an automatic recording print-out as well as a memory system for retaining the ECG during the period immediately following an alarm. In addition to automatic recording, an alarm signal also switches the system from the "monitor" to the "diagnostic" mode in order to preserve elements of the ECG signal normally rejected by the signal "clean up" circuitry (filter stages) in the processing system.

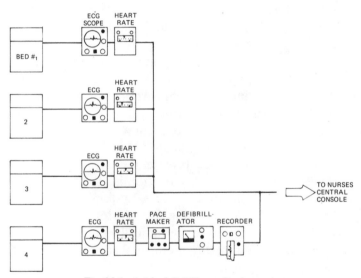

Fig. 23-1: A 4-bed C.C.U. monitoring system

Whatever the size, design or complexity of a monitoring unit and its associated equipment, the primary considerations used in its construction are threefold:

1. It must supply a continuous diagnostic picture of the patient's condition.
2. It must provide adequate alarm mechanisms as well as protection against false alarms.
3. It must be simple to operate and maintain. (In the opinion of many nurses, the "best" equipment has the fewest "knobs," "adjustments," and "gadgets" to manipulate.

ARRHYTHMIA MONITORING

The alarm mechanisms built into CCU monitoring systems are there to preclude the necessity for a nurse to be continually observing the oscilloscope and other displays for abnormal indications. The triggering mechanisms controlling these alarm systems are generally aligned to detect only high and low indications. (*ie,* tachycardia, increased blood pressure, or temperature, etc.). Even with prompt reaction by emergency teams to life-endangering alarm situations, the patient is already in a critically dangerous condition when the alarm is activated, and probably in a more hazardous situation by the time resuscitation is begun. In an attempt to provide even earlier detection and diagnosis of a possibly life-threatening situation, identification and warning of arrhythmia is becoming an important monitoring tool. Cardiac irregularities, primarily *ectopic beats,* frequently are a signal of a possibly imminent catastrophic arrhythmia, such as ventricular tachycardia or fibrillation.

Sensing the duration and frequency of premature cardiac activity (ectopic beats) makes it possible to provide immediate and appropriate action *before* a life-threatening state occurs.

The Hewlett Packard 7822A Arrhythmia Monitor* is typical of the instrumentation involved. These systems require a small computer that is capable of storing an operator-preselected normal ECG sequence (which can be periodically changed at will) and comparing it to the continually monitored signal from the patient. Deviations from the programmed normal information are detected and, based upon the criteria set into the system by manual controls (*ie,* detection of excessive premature beats per minute or excessive premature widened beats per minute), visible and audible alarm mechanisms are triggered.

The circuitry continually monitors a signal from the ECG monitoring system for the R-R interval, signaling an ectopic beat if an interval less than 80 percent of the average interval is detected.

In addition, the system samples the QRS pulse width, continually comparing it with the programmed normal information. If a QRS pulse occurs that is a predetermined amount wider than the

---

*Hewlett Packard, Inc., Waltham Division, 175 Wyman St., Waltham, Massachusetts.

reference width, a widened *QRS* pulse is indicated visually. The system also incorporates artifact rejection circuitry which prevents any pulse indications being given (within reasonable limits) due to spurious electrical signals not associated with the ECG.

BLOOD PRESSURE, RESPIRATION RATE, AND TEMPERATURE

The greatest differences among the instrument systems involved in measuring the parameters mentioned in this section are in the transducers used to detect the signal. The information (signal) processing and display methods follow the pattern found in ECG and EEG systems: amplifiers of various number and design as well as oscilloscopes and recorders. The requirements that dictate any single amplifier system design are, as previously mentioned, determined by the specifications of: (1) frequency range and/or response desired, and (2) the magnitude, or level of gain needed to produce a functionally useful signal. In most cases the type of transducer used in the measuring technique determines the absolute specifications of the amplifier system. For example: a *differential-transformer pressure transducer* requires a high frequency carrier signal for excitation purposes, which in turn necessitates the use of modulators, demodulators, and a carrier signal pre-amplifier. This measuring technique involves modulating (varying) the amplitude of the carrier signal with the detected signal. The result is a high frequency carrier signal whose *amplitude* varies in direct proportion to the magnitude of the detected signal. (The technique eliminates much of the instability inherent in DC-excited systems). In contrast to the modulated carrier method, a *DC strain gauge* pressure transducer does not require a carrier pre-amplifier and hence is a much less complex— though unstable—system.

Another factor often involved in the design of the amplifier system is the number of other (auxiliary) applications for which the equipment may be used (for example, measurement of mean or differential pressure rather than the standard measurement of systolic-diastolic values). The following paragraphs describe typical systems used for measurement of each of these three parameters: (1) **blood pressure**, (2) **respiration rate**, and (3) **temperature**.

Blood Pressure

The measurement of physiological pressure changes is accomplished by detecting force-displacement changes; in brief, changes in volume. Hemodynamic pressure measurements, at various locations in the cardiovascular system, can be accomplished in one of two ways: directly or indirectly. The direct method is an invasive technique calling for penetration of the skin; the indirect method is typified by the conventional physician's blood pressure cuff and calibrated mercury column (sphygmomanometer).

One form of direct blood pressure measurement calls for the use of a **catheter tip** or **needle transducer** inserted into a vein or artery, either percutaneously or by vessel cut-down. A second and widely used direct method also employs a catheter, but in this case saline-filled with an externally located transducer. Pressure changes are transmitted via the saline column to the transducer sensing chamber. In both of these methods—in fact in almost all instances of blood pressure measurement—the systems are calibrated in reference to atmospheric pressure.

With all techniques involving externally located transducers, the size (length and diameter) of the needle or catheter is an important factor affecting the frequency response of the system. To clarify, just as an electrical circuit or system responds optimally at only one applied frequency, its "resonant frequency" fluid systems also have a resonant or natural frequency to which they respond with maximum sensitivity. In electrical systems, resonance can be usefully employed to obtain selective filtering, but in fluid column pressure measurement, resonance is a highly undesirable and troublesome factor. At natural frequency the response of a fluid-filled system becomes excessively sensitive, resulting in uncontrollable oscillations. Consequently, pressure-measuring systems can be effective and accurate only at frequencies *below* the natural frequency of the system. In many instances the excessive response that occurs can be effectively compensated for by incorporating some form of damping into the system. However, better results can be obtained if the transducer is placed close to the point of measurement, eliminating the effects of the fluid column. *Catheter tip transducers* meet this requirement.

Two frequently used **catheter tip pressure transducers** function by way of mechano-inductive action; *ie,* when the material that constitutes the core of an inductor is varied, the inductance of the coil is changed. If a current is passed through the coil and the inductance is varied, the voltage developed across the coil also varies. Figure 23-2 shows this action applied to a single coil, catheter tip transducer. Movement of the membrane produces displacement of the iron core which varies the inductance of the coil and in turn the voltage across the coil. The change in potential developed is proportional to the distance the core moves, which in turn is proportional to the pressure change.

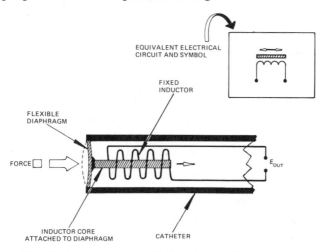

Fig. 23-2:   *Simplified diagram of a variable inductance catheter tip pressure transducer*

Another type of inductive transducer is the **differential-transformer pressure transducer.** Two forms of differential-transformer sensors are common: the dual-coil and triple-coil designs. In the dual coil, a single excitation coil is used to induce a voltage into a single secondary coil. A metallic core, connected to the pressure membrane, acts as a common coupling between the primary and secondary coils. Changes in the alignment of the core cause more or less voltage to be induced into the secondary coil.

The triple-coil type of pressure transducer has an excitation coil, and *two* secondary coils which are connected in a *series-opposing* arrangement. When the core is at the null, zero, or center position, equal voltages of opposite phase are induced into the secondary coils. Due to the effects of the series-opposing arrangement, the output from the secondary coil at the null position is zero. As the core is displaced by membrane movement, more voltage is induced in one secondary coil and less in the other coil, yielding a differential output which is a measure of the pressure change sensed.

Although these forms of catheter tip transducers have an advantage over externally located transducers, due to the elimination of resonance problems and air bubble interference, in a majority of clinical monitoring situations (ICU, CCU, operating room, etc.), the pressure transducer of choice is an external fluid-coupled device. The reasons for this popularity are more practical than scientific in that not only is the catheter tip form of transducer initially more expensive but it is also less rugged and therefore more prone to damage by constant use.

The general design of external pressure transducers follows a somewhat standard pattern. The sensing membrane or diaphram serves as the flat surface of the transducer's pressure chamber which is shaped as half of a sphere. The fluid column enters through an opening in the dome of the chamber and a bleed-fill opening is also provided. Figure 23-3 is a simplified diagram of this

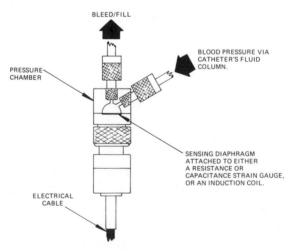

Fig. 23-3: An external pressure transducer

type of transducer in which the transducing element may be either a *resistance strain gauge* or an *induction coil.* Pressure changes reflected up the fluid column and sensed in the dome produce movement of the diaphragm. This movement is in turn transduced into a proportional resistance or inductance change, which is processed to yield the pressure reading.

Other forms of pressure transducers use resistance or capacitive elements constructed into bridge circuits with the active element or elements attached directly to the detecting membrane or diaphragm. As the membrane is displaced by changes in pressure, the resistance or capacitance of the unit is changed, resulting in circuit voltage changes. Due to the previously mentioned characteristic instability of DC-driven systems (drift), a carrier excitation signal of high frequency is impressed across the bridge, and pressure-induced voltage changes cause amplitude modulation of the carrier signal.

Blood pressure transducers, whether resistance bridge, differential transformer, or some other type, transmit the detected signal in most cases to a high gain (usually differential) amplifier system. The amplifier stages have controls for the adjustment of *gain* and *balance* as well as a calibration switch, a range switch, and an overall function switch. The range within the amplifier switch selects arterial pressure range (0-250 mm Hg) or venous pressure range (0-50 mm Hg); the function switch selects the system mode, *e.g., Off, Systolic, Diastolic,* etc. Although designed and manufactured independently, with its own response characteristics, the system's operational characteristics are dictated not by the amplifier itself but, as mentioned previously, by the type of transducer used. In addition to amplifier systems, modulated signals require the processing system to have a demodulator circuit to extract the detected information from its carrier.

Oscilloscopes (in operating rooms) and meters (in ICU and CCU monitoring units) serve as the display or read-out units in blood pressure measurement. High and low limit switches are incorporated into the meter movements to generate visible and audible alarms when activated by the meter indicator. In most cases the limit switches are adjustable so that the alarm-activating pressure can be set to meet individual circumstances.

Figure 23-4 shows a simplified block diagram of a complete blood pressure monitoring system.

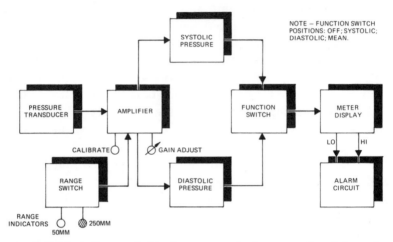

Fig. 23-4: Block diagram of a blood pressure monitoring system (from information supplied by Mennen-Greatbatch Electronics, Inc., Clarence, N.Y.)

Respiration Rate

Many types of transducers can be used to measure respiration rate; a few examples are strain gauge and volume displacement transducers, impedance transducers, and temperature transducers.

Strain gauge and *volume displacement transducers* are usually stretch-type devices attached snugly around the thorax. As the subject breathes, the volume of the chest cavity changes, and this change is sensed by the transducer which yields an output signal. One such transducer is the *mercury-filled* (or in some cases copper sulphate-filled) *tubular strain gauge.* A surgical rubber tube about six inches long filled with either mercury or copper sulfate and sealed at each end, with external electrodes in direct contact with the core of the tube, is strapped around the chest of the patient and electrically connected to a balanced resistance bridge. As the patient breathes, the tube is alternately stretched and relaxed, causing a resistance change which is detected at the bridge circuit. Another method employs the same general displacement technique but, in place of the strain gauge, a *bellows-photoelectric displacement transducer* is used. The chest-encircling lead is connected to a vane that interrupts a light beam. As the patient breathes, the vane moves and more or less light is detected by a photocell producing a pulsating output, the frequency of which is an indicator of the patient's respiration rate.

Both of these methods are somewhat cumbersome and involved for clinical monitoring purposes, requiring cooperation of the patient and bulky equipment. Consequently, the two techniques generally used in clinical monitoring applications are (1) measurement of variations in *chest impedance,* and (2) detection of the *temperature change* between inspired and expired air. Impedance pneumographs function by detection of the change in impedance that occurs between two electrodes located on each side of the thorax (below the axilla). A high frequency, low current voltage (50-60 KHz) is passed between the two electrodes and as the patient breathes, volume changes within the chest modulate the current, resulting in a respiration rate signal. In the temperature-sensing technique, thermistors placed in the nasal passage via a cannula change resistance as the temperature of the air surrounding them changes. Expired air is warmer than inspired air and consequently this temperature variation results in a resistance change at the thermistor. Used as one leg of a Wheatstone bridge circuit, the thermistor yields an output that varies in sequence with the patient's breathing.

The output from a respiration rate transducer is passed through one to three processing stages depending upon the type of display involved. If an oscilloscope or a chart recorder is the display mechanism, one or more amplifier stages prepare the signal to drive the display device. If a meter read-out is used, amplification of the signal is required, after which the analog voltage is processed by an integrating circuit in order to produce a DC meter drive signal. Alarm circuitry is usually provided to detect the absence of respiration (apnea), with the circuitry designed to trigger audible and visual alarms at a predetermined time (delay) after activity has stopped.

Temperature Monitoring

Patients who have undergone general anesthesia are subject to the possibility of developing a postoperative syndrome of unknown origin, a rapid and unheralded progressive increase in body temperature in apparently hospital-normal patients which is difficult to treat unless prompt diagnosis is made. This idiopathic (unknown origin) condition known as *fulminating hyperthermia* or *malignant hyperpyrexia* requires constant body-temperature monitoring of patients who have undergone general anesthesia. It is but one of many conditions requiring temperature-monitoring devices.

The determination of true body temperature has been attempted by means of many varied mechanisms from mercury thermometers to implantable thermocouples and intracranial nasal probes. The sites chosen are just as varied, involving (1) rectal probes, (2) nasal probes, (3) esophageal probes, and (4) tympanic membrane probes, as well as (5) implantable needle probes and (6) the conventional skin surface and oral "button" thermocouple. Most of these methods are too involved or sensitive for general purpose monitoring; in most cases the "button" surface thermocouple or thermistor is used. Of all these devices, the tympanic membrane thermocouple and the nasal intercranial probes are probably the most sensitive and accurate; the skin surface technique is the least sensitive. Why then is it routinely used? The probable answers are (1) absolute temperature (accuracy) is not required in the general monitoring situation; a relative measurement is adequate; and (2) the sensing elements (transducers), in this case thermistors and thermocouples, are easy to apply, involving nothing more than taping them in place.

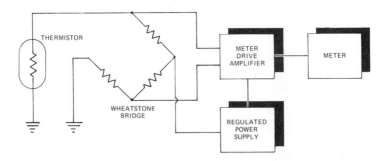

Fig. 23-5: A simplified block diagram of a temperature montioring system (from information supplied by Mennen-Greatbatch Electronics, Inc., Clarence, N. Y.)

A block diagram and schematic of a typical temperature monitoring device are shown in Figure 23-5. The sensing probe (in this case a thermistor) serves as one leg of a Wheatstone bridge circuit. Matching thermistors make up the other part of the bridge. The meter read-out is usually calibrated in centigrade or Fahrenheit degrees, or both, and should have at least ± 1 percent accuracy over its full scale. Some manufacturers employ digital read-out displays, but meter read-outs are more economical, and therefore more common.

TELEMETRY AND PATIENT MONITORING

A chapter on patient monitoring devices would not be complete without at least a mention of medical telemetry. Telemetry, as applied to patient monitoring, involves gathering information from an ambulatory patient without any restrictive direct connection between the patient and the display unit of the monitoring system. In short, there are no wires or leads to restrain the patient in any one position. This "wireless" mode of transmitting physiological data from a moving patient to a stationary monitor requires the application of radio transmission (or broadcast) principles.

Basically, a typical telemetry system consists of two parts: a **patient unit** (usually called the **transmitter**) consisting of (a) ECG electrodes; (b) an ECG amplifier; (c) a radio-frequency modulator-transmitter; and (d) an antenna; and (2) a **monitoring unit** (or **receiver**). The assembly worn by the patient varies in size depending upon the manufacturer; however, most conventional units are no more than four or five inches long by two inches wide and about as thick as an average paperback book. The receiver consists of an electronic circuitry for (1) sensing the radio signal, (2) amplifying the signal, (3) removing the information element of the signal, and (4) displaying the result on a conventional monitoring oscilloscope. In much the same way that a commercial radio station has its own transmitting frequency, individual patient ECG telemetry devices have their own particular transmitting frequencies; with this method, many units can be operated within a single hospital ward without cross-interference. The range of the transmitter usually depends upon many factors, two being transmitter output power and receiver sensitivity, but generally the range is between 20 and 150 feet.

An ECG signal is processed through a typical telemetry system in the following manner:

1. The electrical signal is picked up by the electrodes and amplified.
2. The signal is then used to modulate (ie, mixed with) the high frequency transmitted (usually called the carrier) signal.
3. The mixed signal is radiated as electromagnetic energy by the antenna.
4. The receiver picks up a portion of the radiated energy and amplifies it.
5. A demodulator (or discriminator) then extracts (or unmixes) the ECG signal from the carrier signal.
6. The ECG signal is finally fed to a monitoring oscilloscope and observed.

The improvements in miniaturized and microminiaturized electronic components continue to produce more and more sophistication in patient-monitoring technology. One of the most recent and exciting is a microminiature ECG telemetry unit manufactured by Cardiac Electronics, Inc., of Clarence, New York. As today's Medicare-conscious society places increasing emphasis on patient safety, the provision of an environment that keeps a patient "electrically isolated" is an ideal that many manufacturers of commercial monitoring systems attempt to achieve but do not usually attain. Cardiac Electronics, with its disposable *Telemetry Electrode* technique, is one of the first to offer a unique approach to this long-discussed problem. The use of telemetry and elimination of the usual wiring harness associated with conventional monitoring methods provide this desired electrical isolation of the patient.

Most commercial telemetry systems are too expensive to use for routine monitoring purposes. The system manufactured by Cardiac Electronics could easily change this. A disposable telemetry electrode, the assembly consists of two conventional silver chloride ECG electrodes and a miniature transmitter, encased in a styrofoam adhesive pad which, when attached to a patient, gives him complete freedom of movement. In addition to freedom of

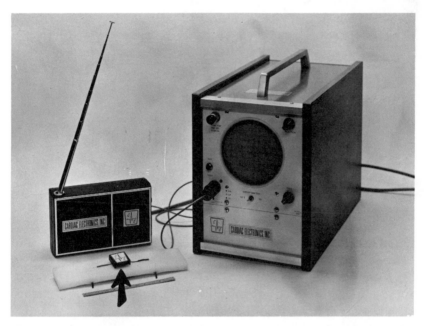

Fig. 23-6: A microminature telemetry transmitter (arrow) receiver, and conventional monitoring oscilloscope. (courtesy Cardiac Electronics, Inc., Clarence, N.Y.)

movement, another important advantage the system offers is psychological: a patient need not feel "wired" to a device on which he may otherwise tend to develop a dependency. Figure 23-6 shows Cardiac Electronic's system with the pad-mounted transmitter (foreground), the receiver, and a conventional monitor scope. The transmitter is 1" by ¼" and powered by mercury batteries, with a total weight of 15 grams (batteries included) and a continuous operational life of five to eight days, after which it is discarded. The transmitted power of the unit is 10 microwatts at 50 feet, and the whole assembly (transmitter, electrodes, pad) weighs less than 1 ounce. With an estimated unit price of approximately $25.00, the disposable telemetry electrode could bring about a drastic change in routine ECG monitoring techniques.

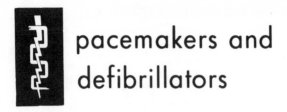

pacemakers and
defibrillators

CHAPTER 24

BASIC STIMULATORS

Physiological activity occurring within the body can be voluntary or involuntary but, whichever the case may be, the final effects are due to the combined reactions of bioelectric and metabolic activity taking place at a cellular level. Although tissue responds to various forms of stimuli, the easiest to study and reproduce is the bioelectric stimulus. Neuromuscular activity can be monitored and tested, and even supplanted with the use of appropriately designed stimulators. To induce bioelectric activity within a nerve or muscle the artificial stimulus must be as nearly identical to the biological stimulus as possible. Physiologists have determined that the typical bioelectric "action potential" is generated as a biphasic pulse, produced by the variations in the charge pattern across a cell membrane which is normally negative on the inside and positive on the outside. The potential difference existing across any cell membrane is due to the different concentrations of ions in the intra- and extracellular fluids. Charge variations in turn are caused by ion transfer across the membrane when the cell is stimulated. Figure 24-1 shows a typical bioelectric pulse.

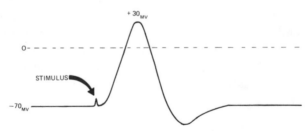

Fig. 24-1: *A typical bioelectric pulse (action potential) developed across a cell's membrane*

284

In order to stimulate electrophysiological pulses, electronic square wave generators capable of delivering pulses whose duration, voltage, and frequency (or pulse repetition rate—*PRR*) can be varied are the instruments of choice. The many parameters involved in neuromuscular action can be studied with such instruments, by stimulating with paired pulses, varying the period between the pulses, or applying trains or groups of pulses. The sophisticated instruments capable of such versatility are derived from a basic circuit form consisting of three functional stages: (1) *an oscillator* or some other form of pulse-producing network; (2) *an amplifier;* and (3) *an isolation* (or *pulse*) *transformer.* Figure 24-2 shows a block diagram of a basic stimulator with adjustments for pulse, rate, duration, and amplitude. Other adjustments or controls that can be found on stimulators allow single or repetitive pulse operation as well as adaptation of external timing devices or components.

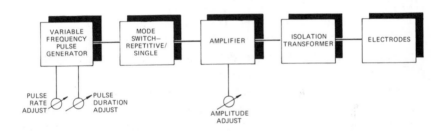

Fig. 24-2: Block diagram of a stimulator

The majority of pulse generating circuits are derived from two popular circuit designs: (1) *single swing blocking oscillators* and (2) *multivibrators.* A **blocking oscillator** is an oscillator that automatically cuts off after generating one cycle by means of a resistive-capacitive timing circuit incorporated into its design. By variation of the resistance in the RC circuit, the frequency of the output can be changed. A **multivibrator** consists of two matched and complementary coupled amplifiers. The coupling circuits between the amplifiers are resistive-capacitive networks and the multivibrator is operated by the two amplifiers alternately switching each other on and off. With adjustment of the value of the components in the coupling circuits the frequency of the output wave form can be changed.

PACEMAKERS–SPECIALIZED STIMULATORS

Although stimulating devices find application in many areas of diagnosis and treatment involving neuromuscular disease, their most dramatic application is in the area of **cardiac pacemakers.** Healthy human heart muscle is normally triggered into contracting by electrical activity, generated at the sinoatrial (SA) node and transmitted via the atrial tissue to the atrioventricular (AV) node, down the bundle of His and via the right and left bundle branches to the Purkinje network. Any impairment of the conducting system between the atria and the ventricle is referred to as *heart block,* which may be first degree, second degree, or complete, depending upon the amount of electrical activity passing from the atria to the ventricles. When conditions indicate a need for artificial pacing, an electronic pacemaker can be used as a substitute to maintain relatively normal heart action.

An electronic pacemaker consists of three functional parts: (1) *a power source,* (2) *a pulse generator,* and (3) *an electrode system.* Although pacemakers can be either external or internal (implanted) the pulse-generating requirements and general design are the same for both types. This section deals mostly with internal pacemakers, and discusses the functional parts of a typical pacemaker in reverse order.

Electrodes

The electrode systems used with pacemakers can be of two types: (1) *bipolar* and (2) *unipolar.* In bipolar systems, both the positive (+) and negative (-) electrodes are implanted into the endocardium or myocardium. In unipolar systems, the negative electrode is implanted into the heart, while the positive electrode is remotely attached (in the pulse-generating circuitry). The hazards that can occur in pacemaker electrode systems are generally due to (1) fractured electrode wires, (2) excess fibrosis at the electrode tip, (3) faulty fixation of the electrode, (4) instability of the electrode material, and (5) corrosion. The development of electrode wires has reached a stage at which structural stresses resulting from heart motion and respiration are well tolerated, with the material of choice being a platinum-iridium alloy coil acting as both wire and electrode for myocardial attachment, and stainless steel or Elgiloy leads with platinum electrodes for endocardial attachment (Elgiloy is an alloy of primarily cobalt, chromium and nickel). The technique employed in the attachment of electrodes is dictated by the method of pacemaker implantation; myocardial electrodes are used in surgical thoracotomy implants and endocardial electrodes with transvenous catheter insertion techniques. When one considers that a normal heart pulses approximately 30 million times a year, the stability of a chronically implanted contact electrode becomes critical. An alloy of 90 percent platinum and 10 percent iridium is apparently one of the most popular choices for stable operation, although some manufacturers use other noble metals, such as orthodontic gold, and even Elgiloy successfully.

Pulse Generators

The circuitry that generates the stimulating pulses in a large number of fixed-rate pacemakers is the very popular *blocking oscillator*, described in a previous section of this chapter. The diagram in Figure 24-3 shows a **fixed-rate pulse-generating circuit.**

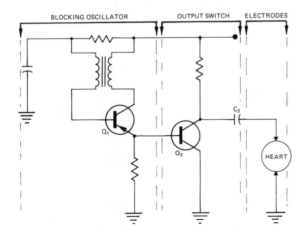

Fig. 24-3: A fixed rate pacemaker utilizing a single swing blocking oscillator

Q_1 is a single swing blocking oscillator and Q_2 acts as an output switch through which C_2 discharges delivering a pulse to the electrodes. The unit is battery-powered. Since the output pulse is biphasic (has positive and negative peaks), it limits tissue damage that would normally occur if a monophasic pulse were used (polarization—electrons transferred from electrode to tissue). This type of circuit employed in fixed-rate type pacemakers gives them the advantage of high reliability and simple design. A strong disadvantage of fixed-rate pacemakers is their potentially danger-ous action in the presence of spontaneous cardiac activity. Should normal cardiac activity suddenly occur, a pacemaker pulse *may* be generated during the critical first half of the *T*-wave, resulting in fibrillation. To combat this situation demand-type pacing circuits have been developed.

A **demand pacing circuit** functions only when required; in short, in the absence of normal heart function, whether slowing, skipping, or total inactivity. To accomplish this requires three operations: (1) *sensing* of cardiac activity, (2) *inhibition* when activity is present, and (3) *pulsing* when activity is absent. Figure 24-4 shows the operation of such a circuit.

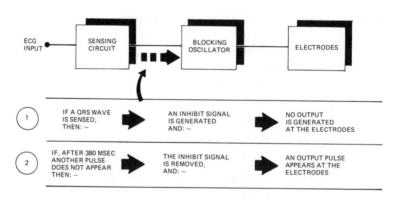

Fig. 24-4: Action of a demand pacing circuit

One type of demand pacemaker functions only in the *absence* of normal activity. The pulse-sensing network in the presence of a spontaneous *QRS* wave inhibits the blocking oscillator from firing.

If, after sensing the R-wave, another wave fails to appear within a predetermined time (310 to 380 milliseconds), the inhibiting signal is removed and the blocking oscillator fires. The sensing circuitry must be capable of discriminating between the QRS and T-waves so that cardiac excitation is not produced during the critical T-wave period. This discrimination is accomplished by circuitry that senses not only the amplitude but also the rise time (rate of change) of the wave forms.

Another type of demand pacemaker circuit functions as a **synchronous pulse delivery system,** producing a stimulating pulse when it is triggered by the QRS wave or at a preset time after the last pulse is generated.

The sophistication required in the circuitry of demand pacemakers makes them more expensive, but longer lived than fixed-rate types.

The input potentials detected by and used to control demand pacemakers are obtained from various areas of the body, including the atria and abdomen.

Power Sources

The power required to operate pacemaking circuits is, in most practical cases, obtained from battery packs: groups of mercury-type cells producing from six to eight DC volts, depending upon the particular circuit design involved. It is interesting to note that the battery-pack arrangement has been used by some physicians to identify, specifically, a pacemaker when seen on an x-ray film, should such an implant patient be brought to a physician unconscious in an emergency situation.

Initially, pacemaker power packs had a theoretical life expectancy of four to five years. However, the body's hostile environment has decreased that to a practical operating life of approximately 24 to 36 months. Since periodic replacement of power sources (requiring surgery) constitutes a limiting factor in the use of pacemakers, the ideal unit should have an unlimited life expectancy, never requiring replacement, or alternatively, have an external power source. Both of these approaches have been used.

Externally powered pacemakers have been developed that use inductive coupling between an internal receiving coil and an external transmitting coil; that is, an RF oscillator generates a signal that is transmitted to a subcutaneous receiving coil and hence powers the pacemaker. The drawbacks of the system are the relatively large coils that must be used (6'' and 3½'') and the necessity to carry at all times an external power pack which must remain secured in a critical place. Problems can arise with this type of unit because of displacement of the transmitting coil, or in some cases, complete accidental disconnection. To bypass these problems, researchers are trying to find an internal permanent power source (an *in vivo* fuel cell). Some of the solutions proposed at this time are (1) *piezoelectric devices*, (2) *nuclear devices*, and (3) *bioelectric potentials*.

The use of bioelectric potentials produced in the body and detected by electrodes has been proposed as one possible power source. Drawbacks in this type of system are electrode-tissue reactions and the low power produced.

Body movement (muscular, vascular, etc.) can be converted by means of a *piezoelectric crystal* into an electric potential that is stored and regulated by a Zener diode, then fed to power a pulse generator. Problems with this type of device have been traced to deterioration of the encapsulating materials thus allowing body

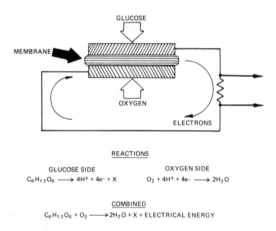

REACTIONS

GLUCOSE SIDE	OXYGEN SIDE
$C_6H_{12}O_6 \longrightarrow 4H^+ + 4e^- + X$	$O_2 + 4H^+ + 4e^- \longrightarrow 2H_2O$

COMBINED

$$C_6H_{12}O_6 + O_2 \longrightarrow 2H_2O + X + \text{ELECTRICAL ENERGY}$$

Fig. 24-5: Diagram of a glucose fuel cell that might be used to power an implanted cardiac Pacemaker (courtesy Professor H. Warner, Bioengineering Laboratory, Yerkes Primate Center, Emory University, Atlanta, Georgia)

fluids to reach and damage the crystal. These crystals have been attached to the heart muscle, converting muscular contractions into electrical power.

The vast amount of chemical energy available in the human body is an attractive source of power that might be adapted to drive an implanted pacemaker. One experimental approach to this concept involves the use of a *glucose-oxygen fuel converter.* Similar to a conventional hydrogen-oxygen cell, the unit consists of a membrane separating a glucose solution on one side and an oxygen atmosphere on the other. The overall action of the cell results in glucose being converted, yielding water and electrical energy. Figure 24-5 shows the cell and the reactions that occur. An unknown compound X is also active in the process. Experiments employing biological fluids have proven promising, although protein blockage occurring at the reaction site on the cell is one major problem yet to be overcome.

Recently, *nuclear fuel cells* have become a practical reality. These power packs are being used experimentally in Europe; the first nuclear pacemaker implantation in the United States was performed at the Veterans Administration Hospital, Buffalo, New York. Research in this area is presently directed toward finding the ideal fuel that will produce good power levels without injury to the patient. *Strontium 90* is one isotope being studied, as is *plutonium 238.* Nuclear power cells generate electricity by using a semiconductor transducer to transform the heat generated by the radioactive substance. The small quantity of radioactive material used (the complete battery weighs approximately an ounce) constitutes a low radiation hazard, and the entire battery is well encapsulated and sealed.

The final ideal device in pacemaker power packs must be able to solve the multiple problems of patient comfort, safety, and reliability as well as low cost. With today's rapidly expanding technology, the only limiting factor in reaching this goal is time.

Problems Associated with Pacemakers

The life of an implanted pacemaker is directly related to the various factors that may possibly contribute to its malfunction, and the care given in avoiding these factors in pacemaker design.

Problems may arise due to any or all of the three following reasons:

1. External electromagnetic radiation;
2. Internal physical conditions;
3. Component failure.

External electromagnetic radiation has been studied in relation to its effect upon pacemakers from such transmitting sources as television transmitters, power plants, radar transmitters, aircraft cabins, automobiles, electric shavers, commercial television sets, and X-ray machines. The most critical problem areas are radar transmitters, high frequency radio transmitters, and automobile engines when the distance between the patient and the object is less than one meter. Although sophisticated filtering circuits can control high frequency problems, the abundance of 60 Hz energy that surrounds us each day can become a serious problem. A 60 Hz filter used to control this problem in a pacemaker also has an adverse affect upon the circuitry used for R-wave sensing in a demand-type unit. This is due to the fact that a relatively high energy component of the R-wave is in the 30 Hz range, well within the filtering capacity of a 60 Hz filter.

Problems due to the body's hostile environment can, as mentioned previously, result in (1) lead breakage, (2) fibrosis at electrode contact points (increasing tissue resistance), and (3) chemical or drug reactions that produce changes in tissue resistance. Research in the area of pacing electrodes is directed toward finding the proper electrode materials as well as the correct material to use for encapsulating the pacemaker. One widely used encapsulating material is silicone rubber surrounding an epoxy resin potting (sealing) compound.

Component failure represents the single largest reason for pacemaker failure, but only if one considers battery packs to be components. Constant research is gradually eliminating electrode problems, and today's pacemaker problems result from failing or dead batteries; few can be related to component failure within the pulse generator itself.

Impending failure of a pacemaker because of depleted batteries can, in most cases, be detected by a properly educated and informed patient or physician. A fixed-rate device generally increases its pulse frequency prior to failing, while demand-type devices stop sensing and begin operating as fixed-rate units. In rare instances some failing units increase their rates to the point that they induce ventricular fibrillation. By checking his pulse daily, a patient is able to monitor, in a crude sort of way, the activity of his pacing unit.

DEFIBRILLATORS

Cardioversion or **defibrillation** is the process through which ventricular fibrillation is stopped by passing an electrical current through cardiac muscle. The high current passing through the muscle fibers probably results in simultaneous contraction, after which normal response to the natural physiological pacing (SA node) unit can be established.

Two methods of defibrillation have been developed: (1) techniques using AC voltages, and (2) techniques using DC voltages. After years of use and evaluation of AC techniques, the trend is toward DC defibrillation. In AC techniques there has been evidence pointing to instances of myocardial and thoracic tissue damage.

The use of DC defibrillators has led to experimentation aimed at determining the *optimum* wave form/time relationship, since the energy delivered to the heart is directly related to not only the voltage used but also the current as well as the chest impedance that must be overcome.

DC defibrillators are usually capacitive-discharge devices using an oil-filled capacitor to store energy which, when activated, discharges that energy through the thoracic cavity (or heart in the case of internal defibrillators).

Voltage levels ranging from 400 to 7,000 volts are used to defibrillate; the specific value is determined by the amount of energy in watt/seconds required, the patient's condition, and his chest resistance. Pulse durations between 5 and 10 milliseconds seem to be most effective and least dangerous in accomplishing the energy delivery.

Figure 24-6 shows a simplified DC defibrillator. The input 115 VAC 60 Hz is passed first through an isolation transformer, then a rectifier, developing a DC voltage that is stored in an oil-filled storage capacitor. When switches S_1 and S_2 (mechanically connected) are in position (A), the capacitor charges. In position (B) the capacitor discharges through the patient. Note that the two switches completely isolate the patient from the power source. When in position (B), the switches S_1 and S_2 are activated by the operator as he applies the electrodes (paddles) to the patient's chest wall, which has been prepped with electrode paste or jelly. Due to many variables (chest impedance, electrode application, electrode paste are a few), the energy stored in the defibrillator is *not necessarily* a true indication of the energy delivered to the heart.

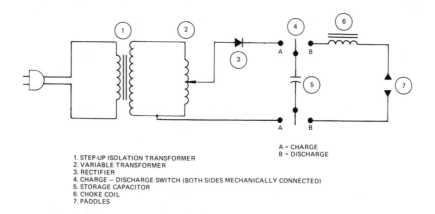

A = CHARGE
B = DISCHARGE

1. STEP-UP ISOLATION TRANSFORMER
2. VARIABLE TRANSFORMER
3. RECTIFIER
4. CHARGE — DISCHARGE SWITCH (BOTH SIDES MECHANICALLY CONNECTED)
5. STORAGE CAPACITOR
6. CHOKE COIL
7. PADDLES

Fig. 24-6: A simple defibrillator

Figure 24-7 shows a simplified block diagram of a commercial defibrillator having an optional synchronizing circuit that enables the defibrillating current to be delivered when a pulse is received from the associated ECG rate computer. This prevents the defibrillating pulse from being applied during the vulnerable portion of the T-wave. A variable input transformer allows selection of the voltage that is fed to the rectifier and hence stored in the capacitor. As the paddle switches are closed, by the operator pressing against the patient's chest, the high voltage relay switches the storage capacitor contacts from the *Charge* to the *Discharge* position. When the unit is switched off, the reset circuit bleeds off any energy stored in the capacitor.

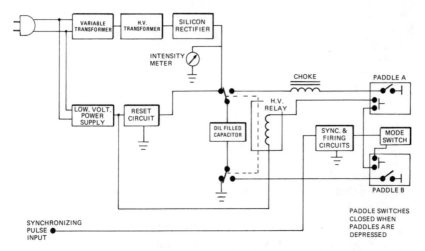

*Fig. 24-7: Block diagram of a commercial defibrillator Mennen-Greatbatch, model
515-904 (courtesy Mennen-Greatbatch Electronics, Inc., Clarence, N.Y.)*

Whatever its design, a defibrillator in order to achieve optimal effect must:

1. Inhibit, fully, cardiac activity without excessive energy output.
2. Deliver energy at a constant level.
3. Have no AC components in its output.
4. Allow selection of *delivered* energy.
5. Have adequate safety circuits to isolate the patient.

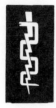 biomedical instruments
employing acoustical energy

CHAPTER 25

ULTRASONIC DIAGNOSIS

Ultrasound can be loosely considered as acoustical energy, consisting of those frequencies of "sound" waves occurring above 20 KHz. Just as audible sound, under the correct circumstances, produces echoes which we can hear, ultrasound also, under the correct conditions, produces echoes which, with the appropriate instrumentation, can be "heard." The unique property of ultrasound, exploited in its many medical applications, is its ability to "penetrate" tissue without producing injury. The process of directing energy at the body and observing changes in that energy as it is reflected or transmitted through the body lends itself well to the much sought after ideal of "nondestructive" or noninvasive diagnosis. X-ray radiology is one noninvasive (in the strict sense of the word) technique that is older than medical ultrasonics, but the ultrasound is proving much more versatile because it is less dangerous than X-rays when used over prolonged periods.

The property of nondestructive penetration along with application of the laws of acoustics has led to the development of many practical ultrasonic devices. The basic concept applied in one group of these devices is that *ultrasound travels through one particular medium at a definite velocity, and through a different medium at another velocity*. In addition, ultrasonic waves, when passing from one medium into another, generate an "echo" in a direction opposite to that in which they were transmitted. (It was these properties that enabled World War II submarines employing sonar units—*so*und *n*avigation and *r*anging—to locate other vessels by transmitting ultrasound through the ocean and listening for an echo.)

This same basic concept of "echo-ranging" lends itself well to the field of noninvasive medical diagnosis. The elementary aspects are (1) transmission of the sound, (2) detection of any echoes, (3) determination of an object's distance by analyzing the time required by the sound to go out and return, and (4) determination of the size or density of an object by the amount of energy "echoed." The following paragraphs will show how this is accomplished.

The velocity of ultrasound in water (1,495 M/sec) is almost identical to the velocity of ultrasound in soft tissue, which is predominately water (1,540 M/sec), while its velocity through bone (3,380 M/sec) is even greater. If a pulse of ultrasound is transmitted through the human skull and the echoes observed on an oscilloscope, the result is similar to that shown in Figure 25-1. The device used for obtaining such an **echogram** may be like that shown in a simplified way in Figure 25-2. An oscillator produces the high frequency ultrasound, and a pulse generator is used to

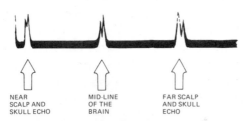

NEAR   MID-LINE   FAR SCALP
SCALP AND   OF THE   AND SKULL
SKULL ECHO   BRAIN   ECHO

Fig. 25-1: A typical "echogram" as seen on an oscilloscope resulting from projecting ultrasound through the human skull

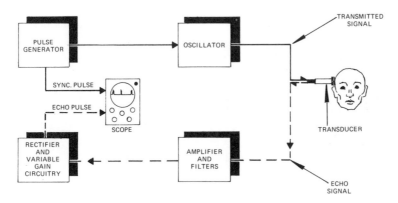

Fig. 25-2: Block diagram of a typical ultrasonic device for obtaining echograms

trigger the oscillator output, allowing "pulses" of ultrasound to be transmitted from the transducer at a preselected rate. The same pulse signal also triggers the oscilloscope's sweep generator circuit so that the oscilloscope trace begins at the same time a pulse is generated. A piezoelectric crystal is employed as the transmit/ receive transducer converting the oscillator's electrical output signal into mechanical vibrations, and the returning echo from sound back into an electrical pulse.

Amplifiers along with variable gain circuitry process and feed the signal to the cathode ray tube display. Variable gain circuits are used to adjust the size of the received signal, automatically compensating for energy that is lost by tissue absorption.

At the frequencies and intensity used for diagnosis, ultrasound is not perceived by the patient; neither will it cause tissue damage. The intensity of ultrasound is generally given in *watts per square centimeter* or *energy per unit area per second,* and is dependent upon not only the *frequency* and *voltage* of the signal applied to the transducing crystal, but also the *impedance* of the phase or medium through which the energy is passed. In most cases diagnostic ultrasound is generated at frequencies of from 1 MHz to 2 MHz, but may be varied according to the organ or tissue being studied. Figure 25-3 is a drawing of a typical ultrasonic transducer head. The coil (*L*) is used to maintain matched impedance between transducer and tissue to effect maximum energy transfer between the two phases.

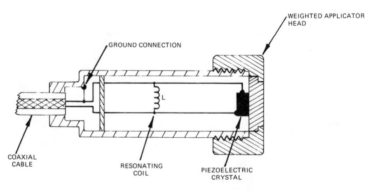

Fig. 25-3: Sectional view of a typical ultrasonic transducer

With an ultrasonic unit connected to a patient's skull and the use of A-scan recording techniques, the first echo picked up by the transducer is from the skull segment in contact with the transducer. The second echo represents a return from the brain's midline and the third from the opposite side of the skull. Note that the second and third pulse have two components; these represent entry to and exit from a new phase. Any deviation of the brain's midline due to a tumor, brain abcesses, or other expanding type of lesions is detected as a deviated or shifted midline pulse to one side or the other. The shift, however slight, is made very obvious when two echograms—one from each side of the skull—are compared. Figure 25-4 shows two such echograms as they might appear from a patient with an intracerebral hematoma. The diagnostic feature of the echogram is the **midline shift** which is noticeable when the first set of echograms is compared to the two normal echograms in the lower half of the figure. On such a patient, an angiogram also shows displacement of the cerebral vessels to one side. This kind of **echoencepalography** is useful in detecting not only intracerebral hematomas but angiomas, meningiomas, vascular disease, and foreign bodies embedded in the brain. Problems in recording echograms can usually be traced to

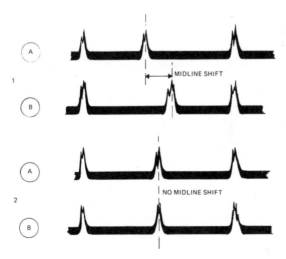

Fig. 25-4: Comparison of echograms from a healthy individual (2) and an individual with displacing brain lesion.

improper coupling or faulty contact as well as highly attenuating masses or increased skull thickness.

Cardiologists have also utilized ultrasound to study such problems as *mitral stenosis* and *pericardial effusion.* Since the study of these two conditions involves a moving organ (the heart) a different type of echogram might be taken. The method explained in the preceding paragraph involved a recording technique called *A-scan recording.* In such techniques horizontal deflection is controlled by a sweep circuit; hence horizontal position indicates elapsed time. From knowledge of the velocity of the signal, distances can be determined. Any movement produced by one of the phases or mediums manifests itself by a pulse being *displaced* to the right or left. Another technique of ultrasonic diagnosis, called *B-scan recording,* is utilized by cardiologists. In B-scan recording range or distance is once again measured by the horizontal deflection measurement, but a relatively slow sweep circuit is applied to the vertical plates so that time now becomes a vertical measurement as it is with a strip chart recorder. The result of recording heart movement by the B-scan technique appears as shown in Figure 25-5. With A-scan, the heart walls are seen moving

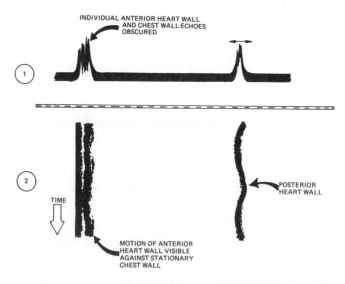

Fig. 25-5: Echograms of cardiac activity using (1) A-scan and (2) B-scan technique

to the right and left; B-scan recording produces a curve that is essentially a graph showing how position is related to time. When ultrasound is focused at a heart with pericardial effusion the echogram recording shows an individual echo for both the pericardium and the heart wall, instead of a single combined pulse.

With B-scan recording, when a narrow beam of ultrasound is focused at the mitral valve of the heart, the result (in the case of a normal valve) is similar to that shown in Figure 25-6(A). The characteristic feature of mitral valve action obtained by this type of recording is the slope of the trailing peak of the mitral valve signal. Figure 25-6(B) shows how a diseased mitral valve might appear. Note that the trailing slope of this peak is much less acute, indicating slow or impeded mitral valve action. Another application of ultrasonic echocardiography is in the area of artificial heart valves. Since most of these prosthetic devices are made of silastic or similar material, they fail to show up or present very poor images on x-ray films. However, abnormal activity of such a valve due to displacement or fibrosis *will* show up on an ultrasonic echogram.

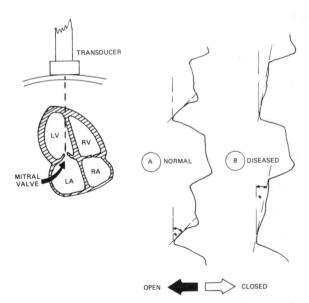

Fig. 25-6: Echograms of (A) normal and (B) diseased mitral valves using B-scan technique. Arrows relate valve function to recorded wave form.

PULSE DELAY TECHNIQUES

These first two applications of diagnostic ultrasound involve rather complex techniques in order to obtain results that are of useful quality. The problem is due to the many interfering echoes that usually accompany the signal of interest when ultrasound is used to study a moving object. An example is the previously mentioned study of mitral valve action. Figure 25-6 shows highly idealized drawings of recorded signals. In actual fact, the recordings are cluttered with many echoes received from fixed or stationary tissue. One method of eliminating much of this artifact is **range gating** which involves turning off the receiver or blanking out the received signal for a period of time, slightly shorter than the time required for an ultrasonic pulse to travel from the transmitter to the point of interest and back, thereby effectively ignoring all echoes except those in the immediate vicinity of the point of interest. Although it works, the technique is not wholly satisfactory, since it usually requires a very experienced instrument operator. A newer and more promising technique utilizes an electronic trick found in radar systems which use pulse delay and differential amplification. In this principle, the ultrasonic transmitter sends out a pulse which is reflected back to the receiver as an echo. The echo is delayed while a second pulse is transmitted. Upon detecting the second echo, the receiver feeds both pulses into a differential amplifier (Chapter 19) which amplifies and passes only the differences in the two signals. Since echoes from stationary objects or tissues are the same on both signals, the circuit passes only the echo from the moving object. This technique has the potential for expanding the use of ultrasound to other areas such as the study of volume changes in the heart and vessels, as well as increasing the precision of its present applications.

OTHER APPLICATIONS OF ULTRASOUND

Ophthamologists and obstetricians have long made use of the unique advantages of ultrasonics. The location of tumors or foreign bodies in the eye is facilitated by the use of echograms. In many instances, surgery for the removal of foreign objects such as nonmagnetic metal (magnetic metals can be removed by electromagnets) or non-metal objects (plastic or glass) has been made easier by the use of specially designed ultrasonic forceps which were developed by Dr. N. R. Brons, a physician in Southampton, New York. These forceps have tiny transmit/receive crystals mounted at the tip. As the forceps move closer to an object, the echo signal becomes stronger and, by visualization on an oscilloscope, the physician can be guided in removing an object he cannot "see" with his own eyes.

In obstetrical conditions diagnosed as potentially hazardous due to fetal size or position, x-ray films are sometimes used to assist the physician in making a decision on the treatment required. However, due to their potentially hazardous effects, this procedure cannot be used at certain times during pregnancy for fear of injury to the fetus. Such is *not* the case with ultrasound, and this technique is finding wider and wider acceptance in this field. Instead of a stationary A-scan or B-scan approach, a type of moving transducer scan is employed, each echo representing a single dot on a matrix that produces a "shadow" picture as the scanner moves back and forth across the patient's abdomen. In order to minimize the effects of reflection and scattering, a water bath is used to "couple" the patient to the transducer. Either the patient is immersed in a water bath and the transducer moves through the water or a flexible tank is placed in contact with the patient's abdomen and the transducer travels back and forth through the water in the tank.

Other uses of ultrasound in obstetrics are to determine early or multiple pregnancy and to locate the placenta.

Still other applications of ultrasound extend into internal medicine: the diagnosis of liver abscesses or kidney stones, and the differentiation of cysts and solid lesions. Since solid masses tend to cause echoes of greater magnitude than soft tissue, a soft tissue-bone interface reflects a large amount of the incident ultrasonic energy, making investigation through thick bony structures troublesome. Tissue-gas interfaces are even more difficult, reflecting almost all the incident energy striking them.

PHONOCARDIOGRAPHY

Hippocrates was one of the earliest physicians to use heart sounds (obtained by applying an ear to the patient's chest) as a diagnostic tool. Consequently, the principle upon which phono-cardiography (PCG) is based is by no means new. Today, the original technique of auscultation is still employed; but the ear is now "extended" and made more sensitive by means of a stethoscope, along with the newer technique of recording and analyzing heart sounds. The former technique is termed **direct auscultation**; the latter is called **phonocardiography**. Each method of listening to the heart has its advantages, and the two supplement each other. The direct method is better for evaluating the so-called "musical" or "non-musical" nature of heart sounds as well as location variances. Analysis of time relationships and frequency components is best accomplished by phonocardiogram. A large amount of diagnostically useful information can be found in the shape, duration and phase of recorded heart sounds.

To understand the design of phonocardiography equipment requires some knowledge of the origin of cardiac sounds. Two types of sound originate from the heart (as generally accepted by physicians): (1) the heart sounds proper, caused by valvular action and being short and well-defined sounds; and (2) heart murmurs, those sounds due to nonlaminar or turbulent flow of the blood causing vibrations within the vascular structure.

Two important factors related to the type of sound produced are (1) the velocity of blood flow, and (2) the pressure differentials involved.

In most cases, the heart sounds of diagnostic importance tend to be high frequency in nature—but also of weak intensity (when compared to the less diagnostic, or normal, low frequency sounds). This fact has been most important in the development of PCG equipment.

A basic PCG instrument consists of the following parts:

1. An acoustical-energy-to-electrical-energy transducer (a microphone).
2. A signal-processing system, consisting generally of amplifiers and highly selective filters.
3. A recording device, usually an oscilloscope or strip-chart recorder.

Various types of electro-acoustic transducers have been used with PCG equipment and three of the most common types are shown in Figure 25-7. *Capacitive-air microphones* (Figure 25-7(*A*)) use a fixed plate and a flexible plate mounted in a nonconductive holder to act as a capacitor. Sound waves cause the flexible plate to move, thereby changing its capacitance.

Inductive microphones employ the principle that a conductor moving in a magnetic field has a current induced into it. As shown in Figure 25-7(*B*), sound waves tend to move the diaphragm, causing the coil to move and generating an induced current.

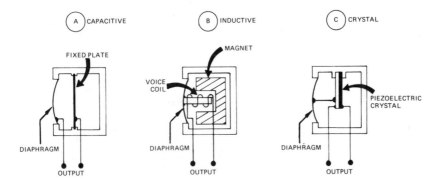

Fig. 25-7: PCG electro-acoustic transducers (microphones)

Crystal or *piezoelectric microphones* work on the principle that mechanical distortion of quartz or other special crystals results in a voltage being produced across them. When such a crystal is connected as shown in Figure 25-7(*C*), movement of the diaphragm causes the crystal to bend, producing a voltage.

Some researchers have noted that impedance matching of the microphone to the patient's chest increases the gain in the high frequency response of some systems, but more work and knowledge in this area are needed.

The most critical item or items in the signal-processing circuitry of PCG devices is the filter or wave-trap circuitry employed. Because, as previously noted, various disease conditions produce sounds that have characteristic frequencies, four or five filter networks are usually employed to cover the whole diagnostic range. The two criteria of importance in the filters used are (1) the slope and (2) the cut-off frequency of the circuit. Figure 22-8 illustrates the load current curve for a wide band filter, with a steep slope and high cut-off frequency. By switching in and out appropriate filters, different areas of the PCG frequency spectrum can be isolated, recorded, and studied.

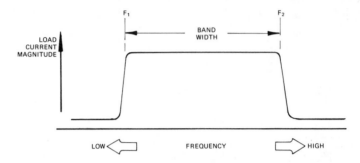

Fig. 25-8: Typical response curve for a high frequency sharp cut-off, band pass filter

The display methods used in PCG analysis are the conventional ECG techniques of chart recorder, oscilloscope/camera, etc.; the basic principles have been discussed elsewhere in this text.

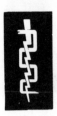 advances in biomedical
instrumentation

CHAPTER 26

No matter how unique or sophisticated a newly introduced biomedical instrument may be, the search for more accurate, more reliable devices is always underway. A few of the new tools being developed for medical diagnosis and treatment are described in this chapter. They constitute the most rapidly expanding class of routine and not so routine medical instruments that can be found in medicine today.

THERMOGRAPHY

By definition, **thermography** is the process through which the thermal image of an object is recorded by means of its spontaneously emitted infrared radiation. Any object having a temperature above that of its environment emits infrared energy as a function of its temperature (in an attempt to reach equilibrium with its environment) and consequently has a **thermal image**. Human beings are constantly absorbing and re-radiating infrared (IR) energy because our bodies (37° C - 310° K) are also constantly attempting to reach equilibrium with their environment (27° C - 300° K, the temperature used as normal room temperature).

With the proper type of detector and processing equipment, a thermal image (called a **thermogram**) of the human body can be obtained and studied for diagnostic purposes. This is possible because unbalanced physiological conditions caused by disease or trauma manifest themselves in most instances by an increase in temperature traceable to either increased local metabolism or increased vascularization or both. In contrast, other diseases such as compromised vascular conditions may prevent blood flow to a particular limb, causing a general decrease in temperature. In

307

either case a shift in temperature and hence a change in radiated energy occurs. Proper use of a thermography unit can isolate many of these problem areas, giving the physician information otherwise unobtainable. A good example is in the case of severe burn injuries. In many third degree burns, the surface tissue damage can make it difficult for the attending physician to adequately determine whether or not the underlying tissues are dead. Thermography, by detecting either the presence or absence of vascularization, can do this for him accurately.

A typical thermography unit looks like the system shown in the simplified block diagram in Figure 26-1. It consists first, of a special optical system for collecting and focusing the infrared energy. Upon leaving the optical system, the energy is detected by a thermistor which converts it into electrical energy that is used to drive a glow tube at varying intensities. The visual light of the glow tube is then used to produce an image on polaroid film. In addition, the electrical signal can also be fed to a special storage oscilloscope for instantaneous monitoring. In most instances, warm areas of an object are shown as white or light tones and cool areas as darker shades. A comparison "gray" scale is used with each recording to yield accurate determination of the temperatures shown on the thermogram. Metal blocks at temperatures ranging from 29°C to 30°C are used to give the comparative temperature data, and these images are incorporated into each thermogram. With this type of instrumentation, determination of

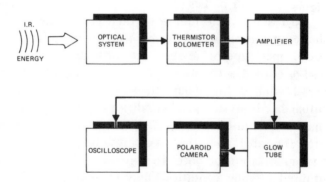

Fig. 26-1: Block diagram of a thermography instrument system

skin temperatures to within 0.1°C with consistent reproducibility is possible. To obtain an accurate thermogram, correct procedure requires the patient to be placed in a room without any heat-radiating sources; the skin is wiped with pure alcohol to remove perspiration. At least ten minutes must be allowed for the patient's skin to reach thermal equilibrium with the room. (It will usually do so at about 32° C or 305° K.) Marker foils are sometimes attached to the patient to facilitate area recognition. A typical unit scans 1,600 times per second in the horizontal plane and 16 times per second in the vertical plane, producing a composite "shadow" image.

An important application of thermography is in mass screening for the detection of breast cancer in women. Malignant tissue has a high metabolic rate; it is therefore at a higher temperature than surrounding tissues, and thermographs taken of women with suspected breast masses will indiate a hot spot in a majority of patients having malignant tumors. In some studies the correlation between malignancy and temperature elevation has been found to be almost 97 percent, making the technique a potentially attractive, rapid, and economical screening procedure.

Vascular occlusions affecting branches of the carotid artery affect the blood supply to the forehead above the eye. Since the same system also supplies nourishment to an extensive part of the brain, potential stroke victims can be evaluated and diagnosed by skull thermography. Thermograms of patients suffering from carotid artery problems show a cold area over the forehead on the affected side.

Some forms of peripheral vascular disease can also be diagnosed by the use of thermography. The point of occlusion and the affected level can be determined accurately from the image obtained by a thermogram of the involved limb. Burns, as previously noted, and frostbite can be rapidly evaluated as to the state of the circulation to an affected area; thermograms are especially valuable when the surface tissue damage makes it difficult to assess the vascular supply visually. Future sophistication in the design and engineering of thermographic equipment will undoubtably lead to its eventual use as a reliable mass screening tool for the medical practitioner in many specialties.

LASERS

Laser technology represents the ultimate refinement of man's use of light as an analytical tool. The development of radiant energy sources emitting single wavelengths of light has always been a goal of the science of spectroscopy. The series of analytical laboratory tools—colorimeters, spectrometers, and now lasers—is virtually complete. The following paragraphs are an introduction to the basic concept behind laser technology and its application in the field of medicine.

Two forms of radiant energy emission exist (Figure 26-2): (1) *spontaneous emission* and (2) *stimulated emission.* It is the latter type that gives rise to laser devices (as can be seen in the word itself: *l*ight *a*mplification by *s*timulated *e*mission of *r*adiation. Let's see how laser action occurs.

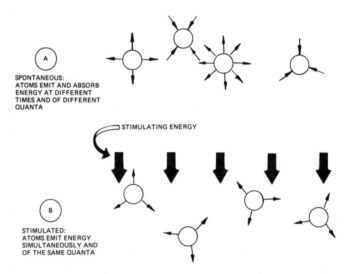

SPONTANEOUS:
ATOMS EMIT AND ABSORB
ENERGY AT DIFFERENT
TIMES AND OF DIFFERENT
QUANTA

STIMULATING ENERGY

STIMULATED:
ATOMS EMIT ENERGY
SIMULTANEOUSLY AND
OF THE SAME QUANTA

Fig. 26-2: Spontaneous versus stimulated emission

An atom can exist in three states: (1) the *ground* or *rest state;* (2) the *excited* or *unstable state,* having taken on one or more quanta of energy; and (3) the *mid-stable* or *metastable state,* a condition somewhere between the ground and excited state. If a substance is stimulated with energy of both a specific amount and frequency, atoms are driven from the ground state to the excited state. Under the correct conditions of frequency and energy content of the input or stimulating energy, a condition known as *population inversion* occurs (a requirement for laser action) in which more atoms are in the energized state than in the ground state. An atom decaying to the ground state emits a photon of energy. This energy in turn stimulates other atoms into decaying, and they in turn emit photons of the same frequency and phase. The result is a short, enormously intense pulse of radiant energy that is virtually pure (*ie,* one single wave length). This is a *laser pulse.*

The laser pulse produced by this action of stimulated emission (also called *stimulated fluorescence*) has two remarkable properties that make it a unique biomedical tool: (1) it is light that is coherent, meaning absolutely pure or monochromatic, and its waves are in phase, and (2) it can be focused to yield amazingly high energy densities at a single point (sometimes no larger than a few microns in area).

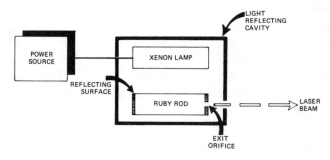

Fig. 26-3: A basic laser unit

One type of basic solid state laser unit (Figure 26-3(*B*)) consists of (1) the medium to be stimulated (ruby rod), (2) a source of intense light flashes (xenon tubes), (3) a reflective cavity, and (4) a power source, usually a set of storage condensers. The action of such a unit is as follows:

a. The power source is fully charged.

b. The flash tubes are triggered.

c. Atoms in the stimulated medium absorb and re-radiate energy.

d. The radiated energy is reflected back and forth in the rod by means of reflective mirrors at each end.

e. The light is emitted through an exit orifice at one end of the rod as a coherent beam of monochromatic light.

The overall action requires just a few hundred microseconds to take place.

Lasers lend themselves to either of two modes of action: (1) *continuous wave* or (2) *pulsed operation,* the specific mode of action depending upon the laser medium employed. Solid state lasers (ruby or neodymium crystals) are usually operated in a pulsed mode; gas lasers can be operated either pulsed (nitrogen-ultraviolet light) or continuous wave (krypton, xenon, and argon). In the continuous wave mode, the requirement of population inversion is satisfied by maintaining the stimulated atoms in the metastable condition.

The exit energy of lasers can, depending upon the mode of operation, wavelength and type of material used, vary from 0.001 milliwatt (argon-continuous wave) to 100 megawatts (neodymium-pulsed).

Applications of laser technology to biomedicine are varied; experimentation with *low energy lasers* has been in such areas as eye surgery, microscopy, and cytology research. *Moderate energy lasers* have been used in both neurosurgery and skin research; *high energy lasers* have proved useful in the treatment of cancer. Other applications of lasers in medicine can be found in microsurgery, vessel anastomosis, and neurological research.

There are various methods of focusing laser outputs, from lenses and prisms to fiber optics. These methods parallel the techniques used with low-energy visible light, and most are unsuitable for biomedical applications, since the requirements of high energy and power densities tend to damage the mechanisms, or the mechanisms themselves interfere with transmission.

The advantages of the laser as a medical tool are numerous. In surgical applications there are three: (1) the beam is obviously sterile; (2) it is also painless when used in the pulse mode and superficially (due to the fact that the stimulus required to produce pain is longer than the duration of a laser pulse); and (3) the laser automatically cauterizes as it cuts the tissue. This latter fact has enabled surgeons to perform surgery that was previously impossible, such as partial removal of a lobe of the liver instead of removal of the whole lobe.

In the treatment of malignant tumors, x-ray therapy must be applied to the total area of the growth to ensure effective action. In contrast, a laser beam has only to be focused on the center of a tumor that is less than a certain size (about 2.5 cm) to cause progressive dissolution of the growth.

The fact that light is absorbed more readily by a dark object or area than by a light object has permitted dentists to use lasers for experimental treatment of dental cavities. Research is being conducted in the hope of developing a small, flexible, hand-held laser to replace the conventional hand drill. Such a "painless drill" would no doubt be enthusiastically accepted by the general public.

The ultimate use of the laser in medicine is beyond imagination. Fiberoptic flexible-delivery probes may someday pave the way for removal of kidney stones or vascular thrombi by vaporization; the possibilities to be imagined are exciting to say the least.

The techniques of biomedical instrumentation summarized in this chapter are by no means the latest or the most dramatic examples of applied bioengineering. They have been presented to illustrate only the trend in medical instrumentation as it begins to mature into a vast new science, and not its specific aim, if such a single aim exists.

electrotherapy

CHAPTER 27

The term **electrotherapy** could, technically, be used to describe any application of electrical stimulation to the body, ranging from electroanesthesia to electrocution (obviously a somewhat excessive amount of stimulation). The basis for such an all-encompassing description is the precept that any form of therapy employing electricity as the main or primary energy source can in fact be considered as a form of electrotherapy. The instrumentation involved in generating the various types of electrotherapeutic energy spans the whole frequency spectrum, with circuits ranging from low frequency, relay-operated systems to ultrasophisticated magnetic radio frequency (R.F.) oscillators.

The least complex electrotherapeutic instruments can be found in the areas of electrodiagnosis and neuromuscular stimulation; some typical examples are discussed in the following section.

ELECTRODIAGNOSTIC AND STIMULATING DEVICES

Electromedical currents can be beneficial to a patient in three ways: two are therapeutic, the third is diagnostic. In some instances, the same generating device may provide currents and waveforms for both therapeutic and diagnostic applications. **Therapeutically,** current passing through living tissue elicits a mild increase in circulation and metabolism of the interelectrode region. Moreover, in denervated muscle, electrical current can be used to excite the tissue, resulting in involuntary exercise. This second fact forms the main basis for the application of therapeutic electrical currents. The **diagnostic application** of electrical currents calls for a somewhat more precise and extended technique of stimulation along with a physician's or physical therapist's knowledge of neuromuscular anatomy, physiology, and electro-medical currents. Such an individual, having an ability to use the appropriate instrumentation and the various kinds of electrical currents it can produce, is capable of evaluating the amount of injury or disease to a particular muscle or set of muscles. This type of diagnosis is based on the fact that a properly innervated muscle responds to various types of stimuli, but a muscle whose nerve supply is damaged or partially interrupted exhibits a markedly different response; in some conditions (*eg,* myasthenia) the muscle response is characteristically abnormal. In general, denervated muscle will in all respects (time to respond, and actual response) be decidedly slower than innervated muscle.

Whether an electromedical process is therapeutic or diagnostic, correct stimulation requires that the stimulating electrode be placed correctly on a muscle. The point of optimum stimulation is at the **motor point,** the point at which maximum excitability can be obtained with a lower magnitude of stimulus (threshold) than if applied elsewhere on the muscle. In most instances the motor point is proximal to the entry of the nerve branch serving the muscle.

Two techniques of electrode application are most often employed in electrotherapy and electrodiagnosis; these are the **unipolar** and **bipolar techniques.** Unipolar application calls for one large electrode (to ensure low current density) to be located at some point away from the treatment area, and a smaller electrode to be applied over the muscle motor point. The large electrode, by its function, is sometimes termed the *dispersive electrode;* the smaller electrode is usually called the *active electrode.* In bipolar applications, two similar electrodes are placed at the opposite ends of the muscle to be treated.

As previously noted, the passage of an electrical current through biological tissue produces numerous interrelated effects, some of which are therapeutic, some of which are not. The magnitude of these reactions is based on not only the current density through a specified area of tissue but also the frequency of the current and the type of tissue involved. The predominant individual effects of current passage can be summarized as: (1) electrode and cellular polarization due to ion transfer (iontophoresis); (2) electrophoresis, the movement of charged cells or particles; (3) electro-osmosis, a shift in cellular water content; (4) a change in nerve sensitivity; (5) a very mild heating effect in the tissue between the electrodes (due to the energy dissipated in overcoming tissue resistance); as well as (6) a slight increase in circulation. Of the above effects (*1*) and (*2*) can, under the appropriate conditions, be harmful while (*4*), (*5*) and (*6*) can all be employed therapeutically. In most instances, the current form, AC or DC as well as its magnitude and frequency determine the full extent of these effects.

Although the harmful reaction of electrode polarization (formation of caustic ions—anions and cations—at the electrodes) can be eliminated by use of a moist pad as the interfacing medium between the applicator electrodes and the patient's skin, excessive current density is one of the most troublesome problems encountered with current passage; care must be taken by the therapist in attendance to ensure that the current does not exceed 0.5-1 amps per square inch or approximately 200 milliwatts/cm^2. Moist pads at the electrodes also help in developing even current distribution as well as providing a means of overcoming the normally high resistance of dry skin.

The currents used in electrodiagnosis come in various intensities, frequencies, and waveforms, and they are used individually or in various combinations. To assess the excitability of neuromuscular tissue, three of the factors important in such assessment are: ( ) the *strength* or intensity of the required stimulus, (2) the *durati n* of the stimulus, and (3) the *rate* at which the stimulus rises rom minimum to maximum. The primary purpose of electr diagnosis is to determine, by various modes of stimulation (emp ying different current intensities and frequencies), whether or nc . a muscle has lost its innervation; a most important factor in the evaluation is the type of response elicited by pulsed DC current. In addition, by plotting strength-duration (S.D.) curves for normal as well as diseased muscles, the ideal waveforms to use in various types of diagnosis and therapy can be determined.

Electrodiagnostic currents range from direct (or galvanic) to continuous or pulsed alternating forms. Table 27-1 summarizes the most common types.

TABLE 27-1

ELECTRO-MEDICAL CURRENT FORMS

1. Alternating—Sinusoidal
2. Alternating—Faradic (square pulsed)
3. Direct—Galvanic (continuous)
4. Direct—Interrupted (pulsed and exponential)

The instrumentation required to develop and apply these currents consists of the following basic sections (Figure 27-1):
1. A **power source,** batteries or a conventional electronic power supply;
2. **Circuitry** for waveform shaping and selection;
3. A **variable timing circuit,** to control the time the stimulus is applied;
4. **Electrodes,** for application of the current to the desired area.

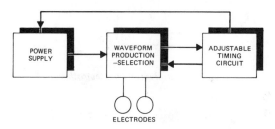

Fig. 27-1: Block diagram of an instrument for developing electro-medical currents

The electrodes used in electrodiagnosis therapy (Figure 27-2) can be metal foil (lead, tin, zinc alloy), moist metal-backed asbestos (or linen) pads, or metallic cuff electrodes. The type of electrode used is dictated in each instance by the duration of the treatment or diagnosis as well as the frequency of the voltage and current desired. A new type of electrode which has recently appeared on the market and eliminates many of the problems associated with electrodes that use moistened pads is a molded, composition electrode of conductive rubber that is thin and flexible and can be used with plain moist gauze. In addition, these electrodes can be cleansed with alcohol or autoclaved without damage. The electrodes are made by the Burdick Corporation of Milton, Wisconsin and are called *Conductrodes.*

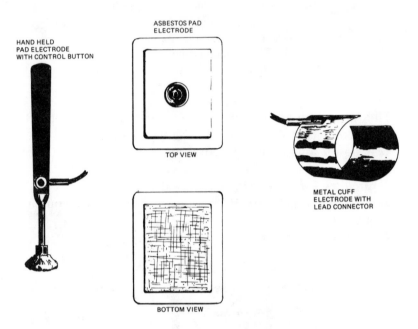

Fig. 27-2: Electrodes used in electrotherapy

The waveshaping circuitry in a typical electrotherapeutic generator must allow for production of alternating, pulsed, square, and rectangular type waveforms. This necessitates the use of oscillator circuits, both sinusoidal and blocking types, as well as multivibrator circuits (Chapters 14 and 15). The controls on a typical instrument should allow for control of the following parameters:

1. **A waveform switch** to allow selection of AC or DC as well as faradic or interrupted.
2. **A frequency control** that allows selection of the AC signal frequency (from approximately 10 to 2,000 Hz).
3. **A modulation rate control** that allows selection of the number of modulations per minute from approximately 6 to 60.

4. **A pulse rate control** that selects the number of rectangular or faradic pulses delivered per minute.
5. **Intensity controls** (AC and DC) that control the magnitude (voltage) of the output signal.
6. **A modulation selector switch** (AC and DC) to control the type of modulation (continuous, surging, or pulse train) applied to the basic waveform.
7. **A polarity switch** that allows polarity reversal of the DC electrodes by simply throwing a toggle switch.
8. **A power-on switch** that applies or removes power to the instrument.

Figure 27-3 shows a block diagram of a typical instrument in this field.

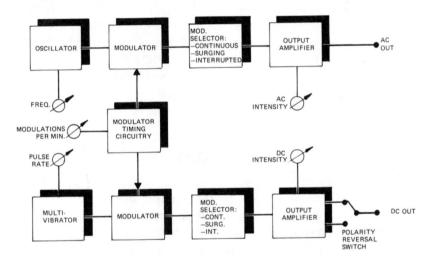

Fig. 27-3: Block diagram of an electrotherapeutic generator

At this point it should be apparent to the reader that the major use of *low frequency electromedical currents* is in applications not for the heating of tissue but for neuromuscular stimulation and electrodiagnosis. This restriction is due primarily to the various problems and disadvantages encountered with the use of slowly varying currents. One major drawback (tissue destruction) occurs because of the excessive polarizing activity (caustic ion formation) that accompanies current densities capable of producing tissue-heating. A second limitation inherent in the use of any type of low frequency electromedical current, regardless of its mode of application, is the virtual impossibility of obtaining adequate deep heating without causing the patient severe discomfort and possibly skin burns.

An exception to the avoidance of DC currents in electrotherapy is their application in the area of iontophoresis. As previously mentioned, one of the side-effects of the passage of an electrical current through tissue is ion transfer. This phenomenon can be employed therapeutically to transfer drugs or metals, in an ionic state, from a solution external to the tissue into the tissue by way of electrically produced ion movement. The technique is called **iontophoresis** or **medicinal ion transfer**. Metallic ions such as copper, zinc, and chlorine, iodine, salic acid, and quinine ions have all been used therapeutically to treat various conditions. The technique requires only that the ions or drug be dissolved in water and applied to the electrode pad to saturate it and the correct polarity of low voltage current be used. (This last item is extremely important since use of the wrong polarity can, under certain circumstances, poison the patient by transferring the wrong ions.)

DIATHERMY

A side effect of iontophoresis is mild tissue heating, but the standard method of obtaining therapeutic deep tissue heating today is by way of high frequency electrical energy, collectively designated **diathermy**. The word *diathermy* implies deep tissue heating, but technically heat production is not a property restricted to high frequency energy since (according to Joule's Law) *any* electrical current can produce heat in a conductor. The therapeutic effects of medical diathermy can be accurately attributed to its *penetrating ability* which permits deep heating without the tissue destruction that accompanies the high density, low frequency currents capable of producing the same effects. The use of high frequency current has the following advantages: (1) it does not produce electrochemical effects (electrode polarization or ion transfer) because of the rapidly alternating polarization of the electrical fields, cancelling each other's effects; (2) it causes virtually no neuromuscular stimulation; and (3) the heat produced can be focused or aligned along a definite path.

The energy fields used in medical diathermy can be one of two types, either electrical or electromagnetic, both forms being initially produced by a high frequency generator or oscillator.

Early forms of diathermy employed spark gap circuitry (Figure 27-4) capable of generating frequencies up to approximately 1 MHz. This type of diathermy is **long wave diathermy** and the energy is transferred to the patient by metal foil electrodes.

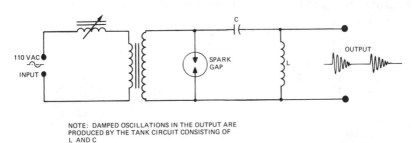

NOTE: DAMPED OSCILLATIONS IN THE OUTPUT ARE PRODUCED BY THE TANK CIRCUIT CONSISTING OF L AND C

Fig. 27-4: Basic circuit of a spark gap diathermy unit

The two most popular types of present day diathermy are (1) **short wave** (10-100 MHz) and (2) **microwave** (1,000 MHz) techniques. Commercially manufactured short wave diathermy equipment operates at a frequency of 27.12 MHz and 13.56 MHz; microwave equipment has an operating frequency of 2,450 MHz and 900 MHz. There are no limits to the amount of energy that diathermy equipment can transmit or the form of the energy transmitted. FCC regulations limit only the amount of side band or R.F. interference that can be measured within a prescribed metric range of the "transmitter."

The instrumentation required for short wave diathermy differs in a number of ways from the instrumentation used in microwave therapy. There is not only a variation in the basic oscillating circuitry but also in the method of energy transmission, and therefore, the electrode or output transducer.

Shortwave Diathermy

Shortwave diathermy technique transfers energy to the patient by way of (1) an electrode system or (2) an electromagnetic field. In an electrode system, the part of the body to be treated is placed between two plates that act like a capacitor. The patient's tissues (especially skin) then become the di-electric material (Chapter 6) of the capacitor, the therapeutic energy passing from plate to plate through the body's tissues. When electromagnetic energy is employed as the transmitted medium, coiled insulated wires are used either as a helix, wrapped around the limb to be treated, or as a flat "pancake," when treatment is required on a flat body surface. Figure 27-5 pictures some common types of applicators (electrodes).

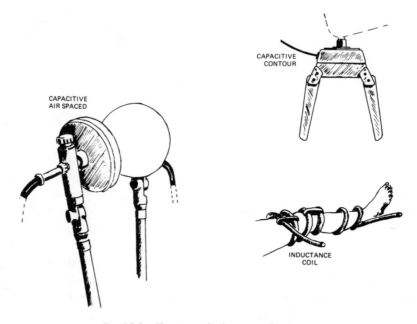

Fig. 27-5: Shortwave diathermy applicators

Figure 27-6 shows a block diagram of a typical short wave diathermy unit. The output frequency of this type of system is 27.12 MHz (the frequency found in most commercial units). The signal originates in a crystal-controlled oscillator generating a 6.78 MHz output. That signal is passed through two frequency doubler circuits ("two for one" pulse amplifiers), developing a final output frequency of 27.12 MHz. It is then coupled to a power amplifier stage and finally the output or coupling coil. The secondary coupling coil, capacitor C_1, and the electrode plates form the patient circuit. It should be emphasized that although high currents flow in the primary circuit, the patient is *not directly connected* to them. He is inductively coupled and hence protected from hazardous high currents. By properly tuning capacitor C_1, the patient circuit can be caused to resonate with the output frequency, enabling maximum energy transfer. The operator monitors this condition on the output (meaning the output coil) current meter (M) and adjusts C_1 until a peak value is obtained.

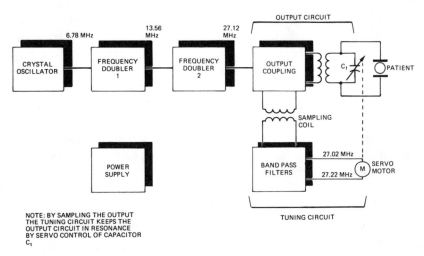

Fig. 27-6: Block diagram of a shortwave diathermy unit with automatic tuning

Most of today's commercial diathermy instruments have the capacity for self or automatic tuning. For example, should patient movement cause the patient circuit to go out of resonance, a type of feedback control (servosystem) mechanism is activated to adjust the tuning capacitor. One such system functions by frequency modulating (mixing) the 27.12 MHz output signal with a 100 KHz oscillator signal. The final output then contains three individual components: the 27.12 MHz primary frequency and two side band frequencies; the lower sideband is at 27.02 MHz and the upper sideband at 27.22 MHz. In automatic tuning, once the patient circuit has been initially tuned, the side band frequencies will be *equal* in magnitude, causing no reaction in the tuning circuit (a type of differential detector). Should the system slip out of resonance (a drift in frequency will occur), one or the other of the side band signals becomes stronger, and is passed by the tuning circuit filters and detected by a differential amplifier. The differential amplifier activates a servomotor, which in turn tunes the capacitor until zero differential (voltage) is again obtained; the system is then once more in resonance.

Another important difference between electric and electromagnetic therapy techniques in short wave diathermy is in the type of tissue that absorbs the major part of the transmitted or applied energy. High impedance tissues such as bone and fat tend to absorb the majority of capacitively applied energy; tissues exhibiting a low impedance, such as muscle, absorb the greatest part of inductively coupled energy, providing subcutaneous fat is less than 1 cm thick.

Whatever form of energy coupling is used, capacitive or inductive, short wave diathermy is generally used to produce a deep, spreading heat pattern in the tissues. When a sharply defined localized pattern of deep heating is desired, microwave diathermy is the method of choice.

Microwave Diathermy

The greater intensity and penetrating ability of **microwave energy** make it the tool of choice for obtaining well-localized deep heating. Short wave energy is difficult to focus and aim, hence the capacitive plates or coil encompassing a limb being treated with shortwave energy. On the other hand, microwave energy can be focused and reflected, and therefore aimed, in much the same way as light. Some advantages of microwave diathermy are: (1) its simple application, requiring no elaborate surrounding of the limb or part in question or even contact with the patient by an applicator electrode; (2) its ability to cause deep heating without elevating skin temperature; and (3) the patient comfort it allows. Some of its disadvantages are: (1) a high proportion of the transmitted energy beam may be reflected by the skin surfaces, and (2) post-treatment burns can be produced if the therapy is not properly monitored and planned. The reflection problem can be controlled to some extent by impedance matching the output to the patient, but only a therapist's constant care and specialized knowledge can prevent burns.

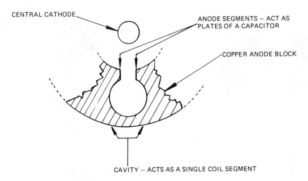

Fig. 27-7: *Segment of a resonant cavity magnatron showing the resonating elements and their electrical equivalent*

The most important and dramatic difference between short wave and microwave diathermy instrumentation is in the type of oscillator employed. Frequencies above approximately 100 MHz are referred to as microwave frequencies and the production of efficient oscillations at 2,450 MHz (the frequency of microwave diathermy) requires a special type of oscillator called the **resonant cavity magnatron**. Essentially, a magnatron is a diode with a cylindrical hollow copper block for the anode, and a centrally located cathode. Multiple circular cavities are cut out of the anode, resulting in a number of anode segments, each two interspaced with a cavity. Each cavity functions much like an individual resonant circuit (hence the name *resonant cavity magnatron*). Figure 27-7 shows this relationship. The cavity is actually like a single coil segment; the cavity-to-cathode slot functions as the plates of a capacitor. Figure 27-8 (*A*) shows the physical construction of a magnatron, and 27-8 (*B*) the magnatron's cavity structure. The device as a whole functions as follows: A *fixed magnetic field* is applied *parallel* to the cathode, which makes it *perpendicular* in relation to the *electric field* existing from cathode to anode. Electrons travelling from cathode to anode are influenced by both fields, resulting in a spiral-like

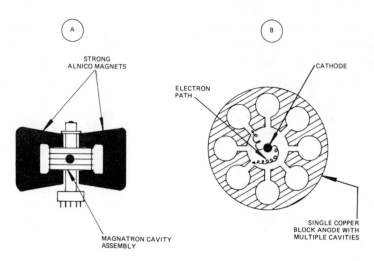

Fig. 27-8: (A) Shows a simplified drawing of a magnatron. (B) A cutaway top view of the cavity assembly with spiral-like electron paths

motion (Figure 27-8 (*B*)). As the electrons pass the cavity slots, they re-transfer energy to the energy field of the cavity, resulting in oscillation. (A simple analogy is the very common toy tin whistle: air flowing through its cavity results in oscillations, producing sound.) The microwave oscillations generated within a magnatron (actually fluctuations in a magnetic field) are picked up by an inductive probe within each cavity and coupled by a coaxial cable to the applicator electrode or reflector. Microwave applicators are usually hemispherical cones or flat-angled reflectors, each designed to allow focusing and aiming of the microwave energy beam as well as a selected radiation pattern (Figure 27-9).

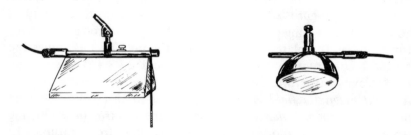

Fig. 27-9: Microwave diathermy applicators

Microwave diathermy can be used in most instances that short wave therapy can be applied. The most general use is in treating lesions of the joint, bursae, and tendons.

ULTRASOUND

Sometimes referred to as ultrasonic diathermy, therapeutic ultrasound is not technically diathermy since its effects and mode of action are *not purely thermal but also mechanical.*

The ability to transmit ultrasonic energy through tissue is determined by the frequency (and hence wavelength) of the transmitted signal as well as the acoustical impedance of the medium through which it is traveling. At the frequencies used in ultrasound therapy (0.8-1 MHz), the velocity of transmitted energy waves is approximately 1.5×10^5 cm/sec. (or 1,500 m/sec). At these therapeutic frequencies, some tissues (such as bone, cartilage, and tendon) show selective absorption; consequently, this fact must be considered in treatment techniques (the therapist constantly keeps the applicator moving). As noted in the first paragraphs of this section, the effects of ultrasound on biological tissue are both thermal and nonthermal. The temperature elevation produced is generally accepted as being due to absorption and conversion of the ultrasonic energy, while the various nonthermal effects such as changes in membrane permeability and cellular functional properties are poorly understood and therefore debatable.

The therapeutic energy of ultrasound is generated by converting high frequency electrical oscillations into mechanical vibrations. The most practical method of accomplishing this is by using a piezoelectric crystal (Chapter 17). Piezoelectric crystals have the property of becoming mechanically distorted when an electric charge is impressed across them. The phenomenon is reversible in that if a crystal is mechanically distorted, a voltage is generated across the structure. Natural quartz is one type of crystal used, but it has a disadvantage in that its naturally high impedance requires high driving voltages. Barium titanate ($BaTiO_3$) crystals are man-made ceramic crystals that can be effectively molded to a required shape; in addition they have a low impedance, thereby requiring low driving voltages. The dimensions of a piezoelectric crystal play an important part in helping to determine its operating frequency. In general, the thinner the crystal, the higher its resonant frequency and vice versa.

The actual transducers or energy applicators used in ultrasound therapy are, in most cases, heavy metal chambers in which a piezoelectric crystal is mounted. Figure 27-10 is a pictorial diagram of a simplified applicator head. The crystal is mounted between two metal-backed electrodes (to which the electrical signal is applied) and fitted against the applicator plate. In some transducers an impedance matching coil is fitted across the crystal to ensure maximum energy transfer. A baffle plate or some other form of backing material is fitted behind the crystal to absorb stray energy. Ultrasonic vibrations are generated by the crystal and transmitted through the applicator plate into the tissue. A coupling medium (mineral oil) is used between the applicator plate and the patient's skin to minimize reflection due to air. Generally, an excess of coupling medium is used to allow circular movement of the transducer by the therapist. This constant movement prevents possible injury due to excessive absorption by selective tissues (*eg,* bone).

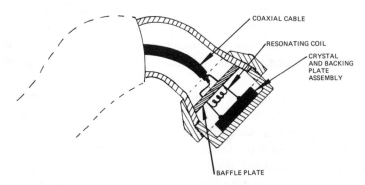

Fig. 27-10: Simplified diagram of an ultrasound therapy applicator

A typical ultrasonic generator might be similar to that shown in block diagram form in Figure 27-11. Note that the timing and adjustment circuitry exert their control *directly on the power supply.* This safety feature ensures that, when the unit is not in use, total power to the instrument is either removed or moderated,

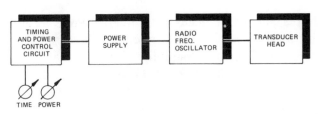

Fig. 27-11: Block diagram of a simple ultrasonic generator

not just power to one circuit. This built-in patient safety feature is not found in all types of commercial instrumentation. A somewhat more sophisticated instrument is shown in Figure 27-12. In

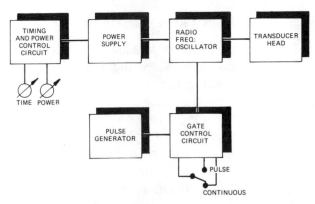

Fig. 27-12: Block diagram of an ultrasonic generator with continuous or pulsed operation capability

this generator, the ultrasonic energy can be delivered continually or in groups of pulses (*pulse trains*). With no input from the pulse generator, the gate circuit allows the oscillator to operate continually. When the pulse generator emits a trigger, the gate circuit cuts off the oscillator for a preselected time period. The frequency range of commercial therapeutic ultrasound instruments is from approximately 800 KHz to 1 MHz with effective outputs varying from 0.2 to 2 or 3 watts per square centimeter. The effective output power is determined by dividing total instrument output power by the area of the applicator head.

Example: Instrument P_{out} = 2 watts; head area = 10 cm^2;
effective P_{out} = 0.2 watts per cm^2.

Small area applicator heads (less than 5 cm²) are not used in general ultrasound therapy, but are extensively used in diagnostic applications (echoencephalography and echocardiography) in which much higher energy outputs are employed. Therapeutic applications of ultrasound are in the treatment of arthritic conditions and other neuromuscular and musculoskeletal diseases.

A relatively recent application of ultrasound has been in the area of phonophoresis. In much the same way that iontophoresis is used to transfer ionic drugs and metals into the skin or mucous membranes, ultrasound can similarly be applied to transfer not ionic substances but whole molecules into tissue.

ELECTROANESTHESIA

The inducement of sleep in humans by electrical means has been studied experimentally since the mid-nineteenth century, following Pavlov's experiments with the use of alternating current to produce the same state in dogs. The resulting condition has been described with various terms such as *electrosleep, electronarcosis,* and *cerebral depression.* Originally the technique was studied for its possible application in the treatment of psychiatric patients, and indeed that is the field today in which it finds its greatest use. However, electrically induced anesthesia is now being studied with many more applications in mind, ranging from the treatment of gastric ulcers to its use as an aid in the treatment of hemiplegia and cerebral palsy.

Electroanesthesia can conveniently be defined as *the inducement of surgical-level anesthesia by electrical means.* However, since some patients seem to show a resistance to its effects, the definition is by no means universally accepted. To produce the condition of electrosleep, an electrical current is passed through the brain of the subject by means of selectively placed electrodes; the current first causes a slight tingling in the vicinity of the electrodes and finally a relaxed state of sleep or anesthesia. Electroanesthesia is still an experimental rather than an applied field, even after its relatively early beginning, due to the various problems encountered with its use. These problems are, in most instances, manifested as side-effects, producing respiratory and cardiac irregularities as well as electrode-site burns and sometimes severe muscle spasm.

The basic technique for inducing anesthesia electrically calls for bitemporal or anterior-posterior electrode placement on the skull of the patient, and the passage of a continuous or a pulsating (superimposed on continuous) current between the electrodes. The electrodes in most cases are nonpolarizable noble metals (eg, gold, silver) held in place by various types of rubberbands. The current wave patterns employed differ with the specific application and individual choice. However, rectangular pulse forms are extensively used at frequencies ranging from a few hertz to as high as 20 KHz. The most useful frequencies seem to be between 100 Hz and 600 Hz, with pulse durations of about 1 millisecond. A typical signal consists of a constant current (ie, 10 to 15 milliamps) upon which larger pulses (5 to 10 milliamps) of current are superimposed at the useful frequencies. The overall current range that has been used experimentally, both pulsed type and continuous, is from approximately 5 to 110 milliamps. The voltages used to deliver the current vary according to the electrode placement and the amount of current desired as well as the pulse forms and frequency used. A major drawback with the techniques employed today is the difficulty in obtaining a sufficient amount of current passage through the part of the brain in question without causing severe burns at the electrode site. This problem results from the fact that the resistance of the intervening tissues, bone, and muscle and tissue fluids prevents all but about a third of the generated current from reaching the brain. Any increase in the operating parameters (voltage) in an attempt to overcome this problem results in an increase in the occurrence and magnitude of side-effects.

A typical instrument for delivering electroanesthetic currents is shown in Figure 27-13. Such an instrument must have automatic voltage and current controls as well as an attached oscilloscope with which to monitor the unit's output.

Before electroanesthesia can become a widely used medical tool, a great deal more study must be accomplished in order to determine the exact mechanism behind its production of depression within certain areas of the brain. This in turn calls for answers to the questions concerning (1) the unique pattern of current that will induce the condition (if such a single pattern exists), (2) the ideal current magnitude to use, and (3) the specific part of the brain to which it must be applied. Although some of these questions are probably being answered by researchers at this moment, once the effectiveness and safety of the procedure are ensured, it must nevertheless then be proven to be reproducible without undue difficulty.

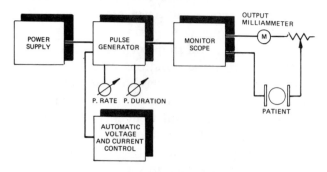

Fig. 27-13:   Block diagram of an electroanesthesia unit

The most predictable application of electroanesthesia in medicine of the future (beyond its use as psychiatric therapy for insomnia) is as an adjuvant (an aid) in alleviating postsurgical complications by eliminating the long recovery periods produced by the use of chemical anesthetics. If electroanesthesia were superimposed on chemical anesthetics toward the end of a surgical procedure, the recovery period could possibly be dramatically shortened. In military applications it holds the promise of becoming a quick, minimal-risk pain-killer that can be used in areas where trained anesthesiologists are not normally available, such as battlefields. Still another use that can be envisioned is as an alternative anesthetic in individuals who show allergy or poor tolerance to chemical anesthetics. Whether or not these predictions are realized, research now being conducted in this area will undoubtedly prove to be useful in some unique way that need only be left to the imagination of today's medical instrumentation pioneers.

ELECTRONICS AND PROSTHETICS

The word **prosthesis** is derived from the Greek, meaning *to place or put to;* and today in medicine the word is used most often to identify a device that is used to replace a lost part or function of the human body. A prosthesis may be internal or external, temporary or permanent, and it may be powered by residual neuromuscular energy or it may require an independent power source. Pacemakers, artificial limbs, and braces all fall into the general category of prosthetic devices.

The single largest area of prosthetic research today is in the design and development of replacement limbs. Of major importance in producing an effective replacement prosthesis is the *patient-device-patient* communication network. This network in all instances involves some type of feedback control (the same concept as found in null-balance chart-recording systems). Prosthetic units are usually sophisticated electromechanical devices that mimic the body's neuromuscular activity by employing a closed-loop electronic-feedback system in their design. The activity associated with movement of a limb follows a sequence that can be summarized as follows: (1) stimulus to (2) sensory nerves to (3) brain (for evaluation, decision, and command) to (4) motor nerves to accomplish (5) removal of the stimulus or some other directed action. By using feedback networks, electroprosthetic devices are able to function in a somewhat similar way. Figure 27-14 shows a block diagram of a typical system. A transducer takes the place of the sensory nerves while complex electronic circuitry performs the

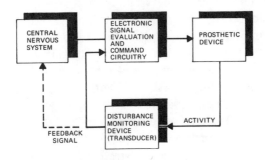

Fig. 27-14: Block diagram of an electroprothetic system

evaluation and command activities, and electromechanical, pneumatic, and hydraulic systems replace the musculoskeletal system of the missing limb. The closely integrated activity required in these units calls for increasingly complex and sophisticated design, materials, and manufacturing processes as well as consideration of the esthetic quality of the finished product.

Although an external power pack is in most cases used to supply the power to *drive* the mechanical system of a replacement limb, the initiating signal source used to *trigger* activity is, in a majority of systems, a myoelectric potential. This is due to the fact that most amputees have some residual voluntary muscle activity available to them. Some typical sources of triggering potentials are muscles of the eyelids, ears, neck, and even the tongue. The most commonly used signal potentials are of two types: (1) integrated electromyelogram (EMG) signals or (2) single motor units. The latter is the most popular source because a single motor unit can be activated at will, and the signal generated is in the form of a pulse adaptable to modern computing type circuits. In addition, the actual movement resulting from activation of one motor unit is slight.

The devices described in the next two sections are examples of some prosthetics still in the experimental stage, but the design features they employ are typical of the many exciting electro-prosthetics being developed today.

A Tactile Sensing System

An all too common problem among individuals suffering from loss of peripheral sensory nerve activity is self-inflicted injury. A device developed by E. A. Pfeiffer and D. H. Terrell at the Veterans Administration Hospital, Little Rock, Arkansas, uses an audible alarm system to warn the patient against such injury and at the same time supplies improved motor control to the afflicted limb. The basic system consists of three parts: (1) a transducer (mechanoelectric), (2) a variable frequency oscillator, and (3) a stimulator (audio) whose output can vary in intensity proportionally to the applied force. An adequate and inexpensive transducer for this purpose is the mercury strain gauge (Chapter 17) which consists of surgical rubber tubing filled with mercury and fitted with terminal electrodes, all mounted within a soft sponge pad. The transducer is fitted to the extremities (fingertips, etc.) and the oscillator and audio stimulator are worn on the wrist like a watch. Any mechanical force (pressure) applied to the transducer results in a decrease in its cross-sectional area and therefore a change in its electrical resistance. The resistance change causes an increase in the frequency of the oscillator and consequently the audible tone produced by the stimulator. The oscillator and amplifier circuitry are of the integrated circuit type (solid state monolithic devices) which permits convenient placement on the wrist. Wrist speakers and earphones have both been used as the stimulator unit.

An Electromechanical Hand

In the development of prosthetic hands, a problem often encountered by the user is inadequate control in applying the correct grasping force when attempting to lift or take hold of an object. Three scientists with the United States Army Biomechanical Research Laboratory at Walter Reed Medical Center (L.L. Salisbury, A.B. Colman, and L.F. Marcus) have engineered a device that allows great sensitivity in grasp control by detecting slippage of the object being grasped and using this stimulus to activate grasp-control circuitry. The system utilizes feedback control from the transducer to the control device; the basic circuitry is outlined in Figure 27-15. When an object is grasped with inadequate force,

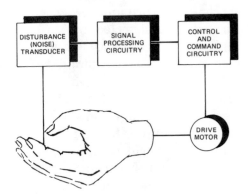

Fig. 27-15: Block diagram of the adaptive control mechanism of an electroprosthetic hand

the noise transducer senses any disturbance caused by slipping. The noise signal is then amplified, integrated, and processed into a motor-drive command, increasing the grasping force. When no slippage occurs, the noise signal is zero and the grasping force remains fixed. Provisions for the user to override all this activity are built into the device.

An Electronic Cane for the Blind

Improved methods for enabling the blind to "see" are constantly being proposed; two typical examples are tactile image reproduction on the back of the subject and electronic "glasses" that transmit signals to the brain by way of a skull harness. A more simplified and less sophisticated but just as useful aid for the blind is a hand-held cane that has a built-in system for warning the user against hazards encountered while walking, such as curbs, manholes, overhanging tree limbs, etc. A great deal of research has been done in the area of ultrasonic energy devices and laser beam canes which employ the reflected energy as a warning signal to trigger a stimulating or alarm system. Bionic Instruments, Inc., in Bala Cynwyd, Pennsylvania, have used infrared laser pulses emitted from a hand-held cane as one form of mobility aid for the blind. The technique calls for three energy beams that allow detection of the relative distance and position of hazardous objects. Three gallium arsenide lasers are used to emit infrared light pulses that are projected simultaneously down, straight ahead, and up. The echo signal produced when the pulses strike an object in their path are detected by silicon photodiodes and separately amplified, filtered, and fed to a variable low-tone generator, or stimulator. The downward beam can detect level changes as small as 9 inches; the straight-ahead beam is capable of "seeing" obstructions that are 12 to 15 feet away. The *down* signal activates a tone generator and the *ahead* signal is used to drive a vibrating stimulator located on the handle of the cane. The upward beam projects straight up from the cane as research has shown this is the alignment that tends to cause least confusion to the user and still allow enough time for avoiding obstruction. Elevated hazards detected by the *up*-beam are signaled by a high-pitched tone. The transmission of pulses occurs 40 times per second with pulse durations of 0.1 microsecond. All the circuitry and components are housed in a magnesium, 1½ pound, conventionally styled walking cane.

The foregoing examples are just a few of the many new electroprosthetic devices being developed today. It should be obvious, however, that the field is still in its infancy and the future undoubtedly holds a host of other man-made miracles with which to aid the handicapped; the only limitation is man's imagination.

hazards, safety, and instrumentation

CHAPTER 28

Ventricular fibrillation, resulting in circulatory and respiratory system collapse, is the primary causative agent of death by electrocution. Since the minute amount of current capable of causing fibrillation (from 20 to 50 microamperes according to the Association for the Advancement of Medical Instrumentation) is outside the perception of the body's sensory system, many deaths listed by ICU and CCU units as due to iatrogenic ventricular arrhythmias may actually be the result of subtle, unrecognized electrocution.

With today's modern and sophisticated instruments finding their way into many "not-so-modern" hospital buildings, and an increasing number of patients being confronted with all kinds of apparatus from external catheterized pacemakers to dialyzers, respirators, and monitoring equipment, every individual working in a modern-day hospital must be aware of the thousand and one hazards that may—and often do—arise from the improper use of electrical and electronic equipment.

A hospital is a dangerous place in which to work, even without the added hazards of electrically operated equipment. With today's ultrasophisticated instrumentation operating in environments having overloaded, outdated, or poorly modified wiring systems, the element of danger is increased. This chapter is intended to identify some of the more common problem areas and the hazardous conditions that can arise, as well as the possible ways in which they can be prevented or rapidly detected.

The two major divisions of electrical hazards can be classified by the source of potential shock: (1) line voltage and (2) leakage voltage. To understand how these conditions can come into being first requires an understanding of the concept of electrical grounding.

TO GROUND OR NOT TO GROUND–THE QUESTION

Case 1: A hospital attendant was shocked and burned when connecting a heated food cart to an electrical wall outlet.

Case 2: A patient on an external pacemaker connected by means of an intravenous catheter died; the cause was listed as unexplained heart failure.

Case 3: A resident died as a result of electrocution while preparing an ECHO-EEG.

Although each of these incidents occurred in different zones of hospital activity, they are related by one common denominator: electrical shock was indicated in each case as a result of contact with both ground and a hot or live conductor due to failure or absence of a normal ground circuit. If any single item can be listed as the most common cause of electrical shock, it is without doubt the recurring and infamous problem of absent or faulty ground connections.

Let us take a few moments to review the concept of ground and grounded circuits.

What is Ground?

Just what is *ground* and what practical purpose does it serve? The answer to the first question is that ground actually refers to earth. (In fact, in Britain electrical circuits are not grounded, they are "earthed.") The primary purpose of grounding is *safety,* and the overall concept can be clarified if we regard the earth as an infinite electrical charge accumulator or source which has the ability to either give up or accept electrical charges without itself

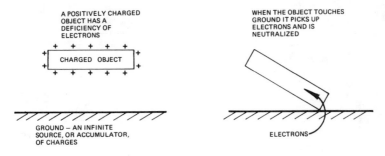

Fig. 28-1: The action of "grounding" a charged object.

becoming charged. Consequently, if an object is charged electrically and in turn is touched to earth, the object loses or picks up charges, becoming neutral (Figure 28-1). Because of this, earth or ground is taken as the reference for **electrical zero potential**. To ensure that no electrical charge difference exists on an object, it must first be connected to ground. An individual who then touches that object and ground simultaneously is assured of not being shocked, since both points are at the same electrical potential.

Electrical ground then serves two purposes: (1) it acts as a zero potential reference point, and (2) it functions as a safety connection point, eliminating potentially hazardous conditions. Both these purposes are utilized in the circuits that supply power to our homes and places of business, including hospitals.

Power Transmission and Ground

In all instances of electrical power transmission for commercial purposes, the power source is connected to its many loads by conducting systems. The basic conducting system is a two-wire circuit having a **hot** or **live** side and a **cold** or **neutral** side (analogous to the positive and negative sides of a DC circuit). Connecting an instrument across the two leads allows current from the source to flow through the instrument and back again to the

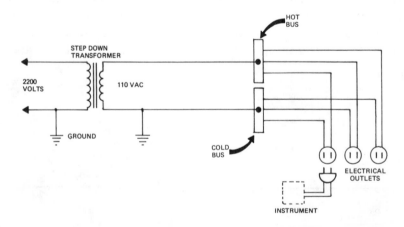

Fig. 28-2: A power distribution system (two wire)

source. The *hot* and *cold* designations are applied to identify which of the leads (the cold one) is also connected to ground (earth). Figure 28-2 shows a simplified diagram of a typical power distribution circuit. The power supplied to a typical building is generally 110-120 VAC at 50-60 Hz, single phase, and is obtained from a transformer that is hooked into a commercial power line. The leads originating at the secondary winding of the transformer are the hot and cold leads. The hot or live lead is color-coded *black;* the cold or neutral lead is coded *white.* The cold lead is grounded close to the secondary winding of the transformer to eliminate possible situations in which overloading of the transformer may occur (lightning striking the transformer is one example). The two power leads run into each building to a distribution box where they are used to supply the various electrical outlets in the building.

Although the major power distribution transformers generally have well-grounded cold sides, the stepping-down of power line voltages to the magnitudes used in the conventional outlets found in a building (110 VAC and 220 VAC) is accomplished by transformer action, and provides the first point at which power distribution systems may differ.

In Figure 28-3, the power for a typical building load is shown passing from a 2,200 VAC commercial line to a transformer within the building complex that in turn supplies 110 VAC (or 220 VAC if required) at its secondary winding. As previously noted, the cold side of a system is that side which is grounded (*A-1* in Figure 28-3); therefore, this type of distribution system is called, as can be expected, a **grounded system**. If the ground connection were removed, the system would be an **isolated** or **floating system**. Except for special applications, such as operating rooms, most distribution systems are grounded systems.

A typically hazardous situation that can occur with a grounded system and an ungrounded instrument is also illustrated in Figure 28-3. An individual who is working with both instrument *A*, which is a properly grounded device (its metal cabinet is connected to a third safety ground wire), and instrument *B*, an ungrounded instrument in which an insulation fault has occurred (placing a high voltage on its case), might happen to touch the two instruments simultaneously. The instant he comes in contact with both instruments, his body becomes a low resistance pathway to ground and he is consequently shocked—possibly to death. If the case of the faulty instrument had been grounded as was the other device, the hazard voltage would have been shunted to the ground since the ground leads offer less resistance than the human body, and current always takes the path of least resistance.

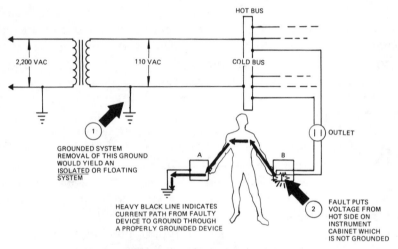

Fig. 28-3: 1. Shows a grounded two wire distribution system
2. Shows how a fault in an ungrounded instrument can shock an individual touching both the faulty device and a grounded device simultaneously.

Grounding the case of an instrument to the cold side of a two-wire power cord does not ensure that a hazardous situation will not occur; rather, it generates an even more dangerous situation. If the power cord on such a device is inadvertently reversed when it is plugged into a receptacle, the cold side to the power cord becomes the hot lead, and full line voltage appears on the case of the instrument. To eliminate this hazard, an instrument powered by a two-wire cord should always be grounded by a third safety ground cord.

The system just described is the basic grounded two-wire system, but, in an attempt to ensure safety from a poor or reversed connection and insulation breakdown, modern instrumentation and distribution wiring techniques call for the addition of a third lead: the **common** or **safety ground,** which is color-coded *green.* The common *ground lead is connected at each outlet to the conduit* through which all building wiring is run, and also to the cold lead (grounded at its source). This ensures that any section of conduit that by accident is not mechanically attached to the overall conduit system and therefore not grounded by that system (*eg,* a section that has been replaced by plastic pipe) is automatically *grounded by way of the common ground lead to the cold ground.* Should live voltage be placed on the conduit because of instrument failure, the voltage, instead of becoming a hazard, is shunted to ground and the resulting short circuit blows the system fuse or circuit breaker, indicating that an unsafe condition exists (Figure 28-4).

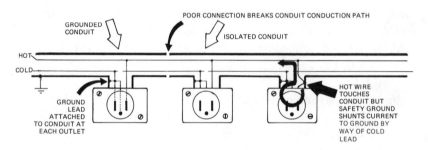

Fig. 28-4: Diagram of a three wire conduit distribution system and how it functions.

In compliance with modern wiring technique, all instruments are now being manufactured with three lead power cords and connectors.

Instrument Circuits and Ground

In the third accident described earlier in this chapter, a resident performing an ECHO-EEG was electrocuted because the instrument he was using was not grounded due to the use of a three-to-two-prong adapter (commonly called a "cheater"). A faulty component had caused a high potential to be placed on the equipment case; since the case itself offered no path to ground,

when the resident touched the instrument and ground simultaneously, his body became the low resistance path and he was
electrocuted. The instrument designers had not failed, for the
chassis was properly connected directly to the third lead of the
power cable, but, because someone used a "cheater" plug, the
instrument ground had been negated, producing the hazard and
the resulting accident.

Again it should be emphasized that the connection of the
chassis of an instrument to ground provides a margin of safety
only if there is a continuous low resistance path to true ground
through the safety ground or by way of a separate, special-purpose
grounding wire.

Another type of ground found in all instruments is the **ground
reference** or **ground return**, which is a single wire conductor or
contact strip within an instrument that furnishes a return path to
the instrument's power supply for all the circuits in the instrument. In most (but not all) cases this ground wire or strip is joined
to the instrument's chassis (ground) at a single point or connected
directly to the green common ground wire of the instrument's
power cord. (Note that ground reference is not necessarily a true
ground.)

In some instruments, in accordance with the National Electrical
Safety Code, input circuitry is purposely isolated from the chassis
or housing and ground, primarily in operating room areas where
explosive atmospheres prevail. In other instruments, the input
power transformer serves as the isolating device. It should be
emphasized that isolation does not in itself provide complete
electrical safety. Although contact with either side of an ungrounded or isolated system protects an individual from high
current shock (*macroshock*), it does *not* offer protection from
leakage current shocks (*microshock*) which may be imperceptible
to most people but catastrophic to an "electrically exposed"
patient (*eg,* a patient who has an intracardiac pacemaker or who is
attached to monitoring devices).

A simple rule of thumb to follow in protecting such vulnerable
patients is to be sure all equipment is properly grounded, but
never ground the patient, either directly or indirectly, through
other instruments or yourself.

TYPES AND SOURCES OF ELECTRICAL HAZARDS

The passage of current through a human body is the result of that body (a bag of conductive electrolytes) acting as a conductor, connecting two points of different electrical potential.

The two most common instances in which electrical shock occur are: (1) when contact is made between two live conductors (the hot and cold side of a power line), or (2) when contact is made between a live conductor (of a grounded power system) and ground. Other less frequent shocks can be traced to contact with the terminals of capacitors and induction coils as well as leakage potentials on supposedly safe objects. The live conductor may not necessarily be designed as a conductor; leakage currents, arcing, and other faults within an instrument can cause normally uncharged objects (chassis and cabinets, etc.) to become live conductors.

In all instances of electrical shock, the current flows through our "bag of electrolytes." The factors which determine the danger or severity of the shock we receive are the *magnitude* and *path* of that current. Table 28-1 summarizes the effects of different (approximate) volumes of 60 Hz current passing through the intact epidermis and body.

TABLE 28-1*

**EFFECTS OF DIFFERENT VOLUMES OF CURRENT
PASSING THROUGH BODY TISSUES**

Current	Effect
1 ma (1 amp x 10^{-3})	Tingling effect; nominal perceptible current
100-500 ma	"Can't let go value"; pain; fainting
0.5-1.5 amps	Fibrillation and possible respiratory effects
> 1.5 amps	Sustained myocardial contraction and respiratory failure

*From data by the Association for the Advancement of Medical Instrumentation.

When the resistance of the skin is circumvented (*eg*, by use of a catheter or myocardial electrodes) the normally high current value required to produce fibrillation across the (intact) skin's resistance drops to 20 microamperes and possibly even less.

Hazardous potentials originating within instruments can usually be attributed to (1) direct contact of a faulty live power line conductor with the equipment chassis or cabinet; or (2) leakage by way of (a) voltage division, (b) capacitive coupling, or (c) inductive coupling. The direct contact type of hazards places full line potential (110 V) on chassis or cabinet; leakage hazards generally produce potentials that are much smaller and hence less likely to be detected.

Leakage by voltage division implies that a fault, such as insulation breakdown, moisture, or contamination between terminal strip lugs, or component failure (usually shorting of the element) might pick off a portion of the total voltage across the device, passing it to the chassis. The value of a hazard voltage is determined by how close (electrically, not physically) to the *ungrounded* side of the circuit the fault occurs. If the fault occurs close to the grounded (zero potential) side (away from the hot or ungrounded side), the leakage is small, but if it occurs closer to the hot (high potential) side, the leakage potential is larger and therefore more dangerous.

Capacitive coupling can occur between any two metallic conductors. (This is known as **interelectrode capacitance.**) As the frequency of a signal applied to either of the two conductors increases, capacitive coupling increases. Conversely, at lower frequencies the coupling is minimal. Because of the frequency dependence of capacitive coupling, its hazardous effects are questionable. However, the potential danger should not be neglected, especially since ultrasonic and higher frequency devices are becoming more prevalent in medical applications.

Inductively coupled leakage currents can be detected in most motor-driven devices, as well as in equipment employing transformers. Like capacitive coupling, inductive coupling is also frequency-dependent but, unlike the former, it does not require high or ultrasonic frequencies to become effective. Sixty cycles is quite adequate to produce inductive coupling.

Whatever the source of a leakage potential that finds its way to an instrument cabinet or chassis, it should be emphasized that if the equipment is *adequately* grounded, the hazard is eliminated. *But,* if the device has an ungrounded cabinet, the hazard is there and, whether perceptible or not to the operator, under the right circumstances it can kill.

THE DO'S AND DONT'S OF ELECTRICAL SAFETY

The following general comments are intended to be a beginning cache of information that will help to develop a sense or ability to recognize hazards or potential hazards that may arise in working with electrical equipment.

The DO'S

Do use only 3-wire grounded outlets and equipment with three-wire power cords. Automatically consider anything else a potential hazard. If older equipment with two-wire cords must be used, be certain that it is *separately grounded.*

Do realize that you can become the "conductor" between a hazard current source and a grounded patient and at times not even know it.

Do educate yourself to recognize potential hazards (cheater plugs, frayed wires, broken ground lugs).

Do replace all frayed or damaged power cords and plugs.

Do use the shortest power cord possible with any device. (The longer the power cord, the greater the leakage current possible.)

Do visually inspect all equipment on a regular basis.

Do use special caution in procedures in which the resistance of the skin is circumvented (catheterized patients or patients in high humidity environments).

Do wear rubber surgical gloves when handling myocardial and catheter electrodes in an electrically "hot" environment.

Do use only non-molded, repairable plugs.

Do provide a single, tested, common ground for all equipment in a single area.

Do avoid the use of extension cords.

Do avoid placing operating instruments on metal carts, metal shelves, or near sinks.

Do look for kinked wires, loose plugs, and worn or frayed wiring.

Do avoid touching exposed leads or electrodes while manipulating the controls of an instrument.

Do recognize that a tingling sensation upon touching an instrument means a *hazard* exists. Unless it is essential to the life of a patient, turn off *and* unplug the instrument **immediately**.

Do recognize that 60 Hz noise on a monitoring scope or recorder indicates a possible hazard.

Do be sure and safe first—not sorry later.

And Now Some DONT'S

Don't use "cheater" plugs (two-to-three prong adapters).

Don't ever, ever, ground the patient—or yourself.

Don't remove power cords from wall receptacles by pulling on the cord.

Don't remove the third (ground) pin on a three-prong connector.

Don't wear jewelry (bracelets, metal watchbands, rings) when working on or with "hot" electrical equipment.

Don't provide the conduction path between any possible current source and the multitude of grounds around you. Either touch only one piece of equipment at a time, or wear rubber surgical gloves.

Don't feel secure after turning off a suspected instrument; it may still be dangerous so be sure to unplug it. (This can occur on a device with a two-wire power cord. If the instrument has been plugged in with the switch on the ground side of the power line, the hot side of the line is still intact and may be feeding voltage to the chassis through a fault.)

Don't assume that because a device is new it is fault-free. Have it checked and inspected first.

Don't lean on metal surfaces such as water pipes, radiators, sinks, or beds while working with electrical equipment.

Don't use equipment with two-wire power cords in the vicinity of an exposed (catheterized) patient. Better still, don't use such equipment at all; use battery-driven devices.

Don't plug in or unplug one piece of equipment while touching another.

Don't attempt to repair a faulty device unless you have been trained to do so. Even then, have it checked prior to use.

Don't assume when working with electrical equipment; it makes an ASS of U and ME. It may also unexpectedly kill you.

bibliography

I. BASIC ELECTRICITY AND ELECTRONICS
(Chapters 1-16)

Basic Electricity. Navpers 10026-A. Washington: Bureau of Naval Personnel, U.S. Government Printing Office, 1960.

Basic Theory and Application of Transistors. Training Manual 11-690, Department of the Army. Washington: U.S. Government Printing Office, 1959.

Clement, P.R. and Johnson, W.C.: *Electrical Engineering Science.* New York: McGraw Hill, 1960.

Electronic and Electrical Fundamentals. Vol. I-V. Fort Washington, Pennsylvania: Philco Ford Corporation, Tech. Rep. Division, 1960.

Electronic Circuit Analysis. Air Force Manual 52-8. Washington: U.S. Government Printing Office, 1962.

Friedman, J.W.; Rice, H.G.; and McGinty, G. (eds.): *Basic Electronics "Auto Text."* R.C.A. Institutes. Englewood Cliffs, New Jersey: Prentice Hall, 1965.

Fundamentals of Transistor Electronics. Fort Washington, Pennsylvania: Philco Ford Corporation, Education and Tech. Services Division, 1967.

Grob, B. and Kiver, M.S.: *Applications of Electronics.* New York: McGraw Hill, 1960.

Introduction to Electronics. Navpers 10084. Bureau of Naval Personnel. Washington: U.S. Government Printing Office, 1963.

Malmstadt, H.V.; Enke, C.G.; and Benjamin, W.A.: *Electronics for Scientists.* 1962.

Markus, John: *Source Book of Electronic Circuits.* New York: McGraw Hill, 1968.

Offner, F.F.: *Electronics for Biologists.* New York: McGraw Hill, 1962.

Radar Circuit Analysis. Air Force Manual 101-8. Washington: U.S. Government Printing Office, 1957.

Zbar, Paul: *Basic Electricity.* Hickock Teaching Systems, Inc., 1966.

II. CLINICAL ANALYTICAL INSTRUMENTATION
(Chapters 17-20)

Blair, E.J.: *Introduction to Chemical Instrumentation.* New York: McGraw Hill, 1962.

Dummer, G.W.A. and Robertson, J.M. (eds.): *Medical Electronics Equipment*. Vols. I-IV Oxford: Pergamon Press, 1970.

Lee, L.W.: *Elementary Principles of Laboratory Instruments*. St. Louis: C.V. Mosby, 1970.

Lion, K.S.: *Instrumentation in Scientific Research*. New York: McGraw Hill, 1959.

Newman, D.W. (ed.): *Instrumental Methods of Experimental Biology*. New York: The MacMillan Company, 1965.

Watkins, A.L.: *Manual of Electrotherapy*. Philadelphia: Lea and Febiger, 1958.

White, W.L.; Erickson, M.M.; and Stenens, S.C.: *Practical Automation*. St. Louis: C.V. Mosby, 1968.

Willard, H.H.; Merritt, L.L., Jr.; and Dean, J.A.: *Instrumental Methods of Analysis*. Princeton, New Jersey: D. Van Nostrand, 1960.

III. MEDICAL ELECTRONIC AND BIOENGINEERING
(Chapters 21-28)

Bellville, J.W. and Weaver, C.S. (eds.): *Techniques in Clinical Physiology*. Toronto: Collier-Macmillan Ltd., 1969.

Brown, J.H.N.; Jacobs, J.E.; and Stark, L.: *Biomedical Engineering*. Philadelphia: F. A. Davis, 1971.

Burdick Syllabus—A Compendium on Electromedical Therapy. Milton, Wisconsin: The Burdick Corporation, 1969.

Camishion, R.C.: *Basic Medical Electronics*. Boston: Little, Brown, 1964.

Dummer, G.W.A. and Robertson, J.M. (eds.): *Medical Electronic Equipment*. Vol. I-IV. Oxford: Pergamon Press, 1970.

Geddes, L.A. and Baker, L.E.: *Principles of Applied Biomedical Instrumentation*. New York: John Wiley and Sons, 1968.

Goldman, L.: *Biomedical Aspects of the Laser*. New York: Springer-Verlag, 1967.

Grossman, C.C.: *The Use of Diagnostic Ultrasound in Brain Disorders*. Springfield, Illinois: Charles C Thomas, 1966.

Light, S. (ed.): *Electrodiagnosis and Electro-Myography*. Baltimore: Waverly Press, 1961.

Light, S. (ed.): *Therapeutic Electricty and Ultraviolet Radiation*. Baltimore: Waverly Press, 1967.

Segal, B.L. and Kilpatrick, D.G. (eds.): *Engineering in the Practice of Medicine*. Baltimore: Williams and Wilkins, 1967.

Smith, D.A.: *Medical Electronics Equipment Handbook*. Indianapolis, Indiana: Howard W. Sams, 1962.

Watkins, A.L.: *Manual of Electrotherapy*. Philadelphia: Lea and Febiger, 1958.

Yanof, H.M.: *Biomedical Electronics*. Philadelphia: F.A. Davis, 1965.

IV. JOURNALS AND PERIODICALS OF RELATED INTEREST

Biomedical Engineering. United Trade Press, Ltd., 9 Gough Square, Fleet Street, London E.C.4, England.

Journal of the Association for the Advancement of Medical Instrumentation. Williams and Wilkins, Baltimore, Maryland.

Laboratory Management. United Business Publications, Inc., 200 Madison Ave., New York.

Lab World. Sidale Publishing Company, 2525 West Eighth St., Los Angeles, California.

Medical and Biological Engineering. Pergamon Press, Ltd., Headington Hill Hall, Oxford, England.

Medical Electronics and Data. Measurements and Data Corporation. 1687 Washington Road, Pittsburgh, Pa.

Medical Lab. Haire Publishing Corporation, 3671 Northwest 52nd Street, Miami, Florida.

Medical Research Engineering. Woods Road, Great Notch, New Jersey.

The American Journal of Medical Technology. Suite 1600, Hermann Professional Building, Houston, Texas.

The Canadian Journal of Medical Technology. 165 Jackson Street, East, Hamilton, Ontario, Canada.

The Journal of Medical Laboratory Technology. 74 New Cavendish St., Harley St., London, W. 1, England.

glossary of electronics terms*

Absorption spectrophotometer–Instrument using absorption of radiation of given wavelength to identify or quantitate a sample.

Acoustics–The science of sound, including its production, transmission, and effects.

Alternating current (AC, ac)–An electric current which reverses its direction at regular intervals.

Ammeter–An instrument for measuring the current in a circuit.

Ampere (amp)–The basic unit for measurement of an electric current.

Amplifier–A device employing the controlled flow of electrons in electron tubes or solid materials (the transistor) for increasing electric current or voltage.

Amplitude–Used in a general sense to indicate the size or magnitude of a voltage or a current wave.

Amplitude modulation (am)–A method of modulating (varying) a high frequency carrier wave to cause it to vary in amplitude relative to the amplitude of the original low frequency signal.

Analog-to-digital converter–Instrument or circuit that translates analog signals (voltages, pressures, etc.) into numerical digital form (binary, decimal, etc.).

Analog read-out or indicator–Instrument information display using gauges or meter dials with pointers and calibrated scales.

Analyzer, chemical–Instrument that performs chemical analyses; may be automated to do sequence of analytical tests by continuous flow or discrete sample techniques and print out or record results.

Angiographic injector–Flow or pressure-controlled pump for injection of dye or solution via a catheter into vascular system.

---

*Acknowledgment and appreciation is expressed to the publishers of *Medical Electronic News* for use of many of the terms in this glossary, adapted from their dictionary and buyer's guide.

355

Anode–An electrode to which a principal electron stream flows. In an electron tube the anode is commonly called the *plate*.

Apnea monitor–Instrument to monitor respiratory activity. Activates an alarm when respiration stops for longer than preset time.

Attenuation–The decrease in amplitude which is caused by passage through equipment or circuits.

Attenuator–A device for reducing the amplitude of a wave. Attenuators are most commonly combinations or networks of resistance.

Atomic absorption spectrophotometer–Instrument for determining low concentrations of metallic elements in solution. Based on specific absorption of energy.

Audio frequency (a.f.)–A frequency corresponding to a normally audible sound wave; about 20 to 15,000 cycles per second.

Audiometer–Instrument for analyzing hearing acuity and hearing thresholds.

Band pass filter–A circuit that allows only frequencies within a certain band to pass through a circuit.

Band reject filter–A filter with characteristics inverse to those of bandpass, barring frequencies within a defined band and offering low attenuation to those outside.

Battery–In electronics, a series of several galvanic cells which, when assembled, produce electric current.

Block diagram–A diagram in which the principal divisions or sections of a circuit or instrument are indicated by geometric figures and the path of signals, current, or energy by lines.

Blood flowmeter–Instrument used to determine rate of blood flow in arteries or veins.

Blood flow probe–Transducer used in detecting blood flow in a blood flowmeter. May employ electromagnetic or ultrasonic technique.

Blood gas apparatus (Van Slyke manometric)–Device to measure blood gases which uses fixed-volume variable pressure sensing.

Blood gas apparatus (Van Slyke volumetric)–Device to measure blood gases which uses fixed pressure and variable volume sensing.

Blood pressure monitor–Instrument for determining systolic and diastolic pressure. May be applied to finger, ear lobe, or limb, and may incorporate alarm for sensing approach to preset levels.

Blood pressure monitor (implanted)–Instrument for determining and/or recording systolic and diastolic pressure. Uses implanted strain gauge or electromagnetic sensors.

Bridge, Wheatstone—Four-arm resistive device for measuring electrical impedance (resistance, inductance, or capacitance).

Calculator, electronic—Electronic device for arithmetic and logarithmic computations. May include digital printer, computer interface.

Cannula—Tube or needle for insertion into body.

Calibration—The process of comparing an instrument or device with a standard to determine its accuracy or to devise a corrected scale.

Capacitance—The property of a capacitor (condenser) which determines the amount of electrical energy which can be stored in it by applying a given voltage.

Capacitive coupling—That type of interconnection between stages of an amplifier which employs a capacitor in the circuit between the plate of one tube and the grid of the succeeding one (collector to base in transistor circuits).

Capacitor—Two or more conductors separated by a nonconductor (dielectric) such as glass, paper, air, oil, or mica. Used to store electrical energy (same function as *condenser*).

Cardiac monitor—Instrument that gives an oscilloscope display of heart wave. Combines features of several cardiac instruments such as electrocardiograph, cardiotachometer, etc.; it may also allow upper and lower limits to be set and trigger audible and/or visual alarms when limits are exceeded.

Cardiac pacemaker—Device that stimulates the heart to contract. Controls its rhythm by means of electrodes placed on the chest wall or implanted into the heart muscle.

Carrier—A high frequency wave which may be marked or modulated either by changing its amplitude, frequency, or phase so that it may "carry" intelligence.

Catheter—Tube for injecting or withdrawing fluid or for inserting electrode into vein or artery.

Cathode—In an electron tube, the electrode from which the electrons are emitted.

Cathode-ray tube—An electron tube in which a beam of electrons is used to reproduce an image on its flourescent screen.

Cell, ultraviolet—Cell for use in analysis of high absorbance samples in UV and visible light.

Centrifuge—Rotating machine using centrifugal force for separating constituents of a solution, mixture, or suspension according to their specific gravity or weight.

Charge—The electrical energy stored in a capacitor or battery or held on an insulated object.

Chassis—The framework on which the parts of electronic equipment are mounted.

Chloridimeter (chloridometer)—Instrument for measuring chloride content of blood serum, urine or other biological fluids.

Choke coil—A coil which allows direct current to pass but retards alternating current.

Chromatograph—Apparatus for analysis of chemicals and compounds by their affinity to adsorbents, as in a separation column using adsorption techniques. Types include gas, liquid, paper, thin layer.

Chronaximeter (chronomyometer)—Instrument for measurement of time required for a stimulus to excite a nerve element.

Circuit—A connected assemblage of electrical components such as resistors, capacitors, and inductors having desired electrical characteristics.

Clot timer: coagulation timer—Instrument that measures time required for blood plasma to coagulate or clot. Indicates fibrin content.

Colorimeter—Photoelectric instrument for measuring color differences or colors. Basic analytical instrument for analysis of chemical compounds and solutions by colorimetric technique.

Computer, analog—Electronic computer which simulates parameters (temperature, pressure, flow, etc.) by analogous electrical signals (voltage); electronic differential analyzer; computer using analog techniques, such as operational-amplifier integrators, to stimulate and solve equations expressed in integral or differential forms.

Computer, digital—Electronic calculating machine which calculates by discrete numerical techniques, usually using binary arithmetic techniques, and featuring a "memory" for data input, output, and arithmetic units.

Condenser—See *Capacitor*

Conductance—The relative ease with which a conductor transmits electrical energy. The reciprocal or resistance.

Conductor—A medium capable of carrying an electric current, usually a metallic wire.

Counter, blood cell—Device that counts number of leukocytes (white blood cells) and erythrocytes (red blood cells) in blood.

Counter, Geiger-Muller—Gas chamber type radiation counter in which chamber operates in avalanche region for high amplification and sensitivity.

Counter, radiation—Device for counting radiation particles (alpha, beta, gamma, neutrons, etc.) or photons of energy (x-ray, etc.) usually using either scintillation or ionization resulting from presence of particle or photon to be measured.

Counter, scintillation—Type of radiation counter in which incoming particles or photons are counted by means of scintillation induced when the incident radiation strikes a crystal phosphor. A photomultiplier is used for detecting and amplifying photons produced by incident ionizing radiation, within the crystal.

Coupling—The connection between two circuits that enables electrical energy or signals to be transferred from one to the other.

Crystal (Xtal)—A material, usually natural quartz, which vibrates at a fixed frequency, depending on its size. Used to maintain accurate frequency and stability.

Current-leak detector—Device that indicates leakage current in electrical equipment.

Cycle—A unit in a wave pattern that recurs at regular intervals. The number of cycles occurring in one second (cps, Hz) of the frequency.

Damping—The loss of energy in a mechanical or electrical system by dissipation, absorption or radiation.

Defibrillator—Device used to eliminate fibrillation (irregular beating) of the heart muscle by application of high voltage impulses.

Demodulation—The process of extracting the signal intelligence from a modulated carrier wave. Also called *detection*.

Detector, thermal conductivity—Device for indicating heat flux through metal, gas, solution, etc.

Dialyzer, dialysis apparatus, hemodialyzer—Apparatus for separating crystals and colloids in blood or some other fluid using a semipermeable membrane.

Diffraction grating—Series of closely spaced parallel lines or reflecting surfaces which produce a spectrum of incident radiation.

Digital integrator—Device for summing or totalizing areas under curves. Gives numerical readout.

Digital readout indicator—Display that reads directly in numerical form, as opposed to analog indicator needle and scale.

Digital-to-analog converter—Device that changes a digital signal (binary, decimal, etc.) into its analog equivalent (voltage or current).

Diode—An electron tube with two electrodes, a cathode and an anode. Principally used (1) to convert alternating currents to pulsating current and (2) as a detector.

Direct current (DC, dc)—Electric current flowing through a circuit in one direction.

Distortion—Usually a change of wave form. More commonly used to describe a degradation of wave form.

ECG, EKG—Abbreviation for electrocardiograph, electrocardiography and electrocardiogram. See *Electrocardiograph.*

Echoencephalograph—Device using ultrasonic energy and echo-ranging technique to determine brain midline, hematomas, tumor.

Electric field—The region around an electrically charged body wherein lines of electric stress exist.

Electric shield—A housing of metal, usually aluminum or copper, placed around a circuit. Provides a low-resistance or ground for high-frequency radiations.

Electricity—A fundamental quantity in nature consisting of elementary particles: electrons (negative) and positrons (positive).

Electrocardiograph (ECG)—Instrument that measures and records electrical potentials generated at the body surface during contraction and relaxation of the heart muscle.

Electrocardiophonograph—Instrument that records heart sounds.

Electrode (as used in electronics)—In an electron tube, the conducting element that performs one or more of the functions of emitting, collecting, or controlling electrons. Electrodes include *cathodes, grids, plates.*

Electrode (as used in medical applications)—Terminal connecting a conventional conductor (wire) to an object, body, or electric circuit; poles of a battery. Positive electrode is called *anode;* negative electrode is called *cathode.*

Electrode, blood gas—Electrode for determining PO_2 and PCO_2 in blood. Uses selectively permeable membranes or electromagnetic techniques.

Electrode, ECG—In unipolar ECG, the active (exploring) electrode is on chest near heart and is used with a remote (indifferent) electrode on limb. When three or four limbs are used, they are joined to form a central electrode which becomes the "indifferent" electrode. Usually silver-silver chloride metal.

Electrode, EEG—Electrode that attaches to scalp for detecting brain waves.

Electrode, EMG—Electrode for use in muscle studies.

Electrode, needle—Used for subcutaneous electrical recording and stimulating.

Electrode, pH—Sensor comprising thin-walled glass membrane (glass electrode) or spongy platinum exposed to gaseous hydrogen (hydrogen electrode) or platinum exposed to quinhydron (quinhydrone electrode), all of which develop an electric force proportional to the hydrogen-ion activity of a solution when immersed in the solution.

Electroencephalograph (EEG)—Instrument for measuring and recording potentials produced by the brain.

Electroencephaloscope—Instrument for detecting brain potentials at many different sections of brain and displaying them on a cathode-ray tube.

Electrolyte—A liquid, chemical paste, or similar material which forms a conducting medium.

Electromagnetic field—A magnetic field resulting from the flow of electricity.

Electrometer, vacuum tube—A vacuum tube amplifier with very high input impedance.

Electromyograph (EMG)—Instrument for measuring and recording potentials generated by muscles.

Electron gun—That portion of a cathode-ray tube which emits a beam of controlled electrons.

Electron tube—A highly evacuated or gas-filled tube in which electrons are emitted and controlled.

Electronic—Of or pertaining to apparatus utilizing electron devices.

Electrophoresis apparatus—Apparatus for producing migration of charged particles (ions) in solution in an electric field. Basically a constant voltage or constant current power supply with electrodes. Types include paper, cascading electrodes, high voltage, gel, thin layer.

Emission secondary—The liberation of electrons from an element within a tube other than the cathode, due to impact of high velocity electrons.

Emission, thermionic—The liberation of electrons due to the temperature rise of a cathode alone, independent of any other electrodes within the tube.

Farad—The basic unit of capacitance.

Feedback—Regeneration (positive feedback) or degeneration (negative feedback) involving coupling from a high level point in an amplifier to a lower level point in the same or a previous stage in such a manner as either to increase or to decrease the apparent gain of the amplifier.

Fiber optics probe—Flexible probe made up of a bundle of fine glass fibers optically aligned to transmit image, transmit light or both.

Filter, electrical—A network of reactive elements so arranged as to exhibit frequency-discriminating characteristics.

Filter, optical—Device for passing or rejecting a specific spectrum or wavelength of optical radiation.

Flowmeter, magnetic—Flowmeter using electromagnetic principle as fluid stream (*ie,* blood) passes through coil around flow passage (artery or vein) to measure flow rate.

Fluorometer—Instrument for measuring ultraviolet radiation. Causes fluorescence in a sample.

Gain—The ratio of output to input voltage, current or power. Usually expressed in decibles.

Galvanometer—Highly sensitive instrument for measuring small currents by electromagnetic reaction. Usually a movable coil in field of a permanent magnet (D'Arsonval movement) or a thread of platinum between poles of a strong magnet (Einthoven string galvanometer). Lightbeam galvanometer has mirror on movable element so that position of element is indicated by position or spot of light reflected from mirror.

Gas analyzer—Analytical instrument for determining composition of a gas.

Gas tube—An evacuated electron tube with a small amount of gas sealed inside. Ionization of the gas molecules during operation is responsible for the current flow.

Geiger-Muller counter—Radiation counter tube, usually a gas-filled cylinder with concentric wire held at a positive potential with respect to the cylinder. An ionizing particle or ray produces ions in the gas which in turn create a uniform-amplitude voltage pulse between the electrodes, independent of the energy of the initial ionizing agent.

Grid—An electrode having one or more openings, placed between the cathode and anode in an electron tube to control the flow of electrons from cathode to anode.

Heater—An element in an electron tube which indirectly heats the cathode.

Henry—The basic unit of inductance. (plural: henrys)

High-pass filter—A filter which passes all frequencies above a certain point, and attenuates all frequencies below that point.

Impedance—That property of an electrical circuit which opposes the flow of alternating current.

Impedance matching—A method of minimizing the adverse effects of junctions between dissimilar circuits.

Inductance—That property of a coil or circuit which causes current changes to lag behind voltage changes. Measured in henrys.

Infrared detector—Transducer which is sensitive to infrared radiation (wavelength between 0.75 and 1,000 microns). Usually uses a semiconductor, thermocouple, bolometer or pneumatic (pressure) device to detect the radiation.

Infrared sources—Emitters of radiation with wavelength between 0.75 and 1,000 microns.

Inhalation therapy equipment—Inhalators, thoracic suction equipment, vacuum pumps, emergency (resuscitation) equipment used to assist patient respiration or administer therapy via vapor.

Interference—Disturbance in electrical circuits caused by undesired signals, stray currents, poor grounds, etc.

Ionization—The conversion of gas molecules into ions through the loss or gain of electrons.

Ionization chamber—Chamber with small amount of gas, across which an electric gradient can be applied. (An ionizing event ionizes the gas.)

Iontophoresis apparatus—Device which uses electric current to analyze a solution as its ions separate in an electric field. Also used to introduce ions of soluble salts into body tissues.

Kilo—A prefix meaning one thousand (*eg,* kilovolt).

Laser—Light Amplification by Stimulated Emission of Radiation. Device for amplifying or modulating a light beam by stimulating the emission of coherent (same wavelength, same phase) radiation from a gas, liquid or solid.

Light source—Illuminator. Many types available, all based on wavelength required; carbon arc, deuterium, flashing light, hollow cathode, hydrogen, infrared mercury, sodium, spectra, stroboscope, ultraviolet, zirconium, xenon.

Load—(1) The power consumed by a machine or circuit in performing its function. (2) A power-consuming device connected to a circuit.

Loss—The amount of electrical attenuation in a circuit, or the power consumed in a circuit component.

Low pass-filter—A filter network which passes all frequencies below a specified frequency with little or no loss but which discriminates strongly against higher frequencies.

Magnetron—An electron tube in which the path of an electron beam is determined by an external magnetic field. Used in ultrahigh frequency applications.

Mass spectrometer—Analytical instrument which identifies a substance by deflecting a stream of electrified particles (ions) according to their mass. When stream of charged particles enters a magnetic field, it is deflected into a semicircular path, ultimately striking a photographic plate or photomultiplier tube sensor.

Matching—Coupling two circuits so that energy can be transferred from one to the other with minimum loss.

Megacycle (mc)—One million cycles.

Megohm (meg)—One million ohms.

Micro—A prefix meaning one millionth (*eg,* microvolt)

Milli—A prefix meaning one thousandth (*eg,* millisecond, milliampere).

Monitor, patient physiological—Device for automatically measuring and/or recording one or several physiological parameters, including heart potential, blood flow, blood pressure, pulse rate, temperature, etc.

Monochromator—Device for isolating and transmitting light of a single wavelength.

Noise—Any unintelligible signals in a system which tend to interfere with the desired signals.

Ohm—Basic unit of electrical resistance, equivalent to that resistance in which a current of one ampere can be maintained by a potential of one volt.

Open circuit—An electrical circuit that is broken or interrupted.

Oscillator—An electronic device which generates alternating-current power at a frequency determined by the values of certain constants in its circuits.

Oscilloscope—An apparatus embodying a cathode ray tube which produces instantaneously a continuous display representing the values of a rapidly varying electrical quantity.

Pentode–Electron tube with five electrodes: a cathode (electron emitter), a plate (electron collector), and three grids (controlling the flow of electrons).

Phase angle–The difference in phase between corresponding points in two or more cyclic operations. Expressed in degrees.

pH electrode–Transducer sensitive to hydrogen ion activity.

pH meter–Instrument for measuring hydrogen-ion activity of a solution. Basically a high input impedance voltmeter.

Phonocardiograph–Instrument for recording sounds of the heart on a strip chart recorder.

Phonoelectrocardioscope–Dual-beam oscilloscope which displays both ECG signals and heart sound signals simultaneously.

Photocell–Device which indicates intensity of light incident upon it by some electrical characteristic, usually a voltage generated or resistance change. The electrical properties of the cell are affected by light.

Photoelectric emission–The emission of electrons from certain materials when exposed to light.

Photometer–Device for measuring light intensity.

Photometer, flame–Analytical instrument using light emitted by substance in a flame. Commonly used for determination of sodium, potassium, and calcium in biological materials.

Phototube–An electron tube in which variations in applied light cause corresponding variations in electron emission.

Piezoelectric effect–That property of certain natural and synthetic crystals by which they are mechanically deformed under the influence of an electric field (and vice versa).

Plethysmograph–Device that measures change in volume of tissue, organ, or body resulting from changing quantity of blood. Transducers used are strain gauges or photocells.

Pneumotachygraph–Measures velocity of respired air, breathing rate.

Potential–The difference in voltage between two points.

Preamplifier–Amplifier used to increase power of weak signals, as from transducers.

Pressure transducer–Device for converting pressure pulsations into electric signals. Commonly strain gauges or electromagnetic.

Probe–Small device for subcutaneous or surface examination or stimulation.

Pulse–A surge of electrical energy of short duration.

Radiation–Electromagnetic energy traveling in space, such as light, radio waves, infrared waves, x-rays, etc.

Ratemeter, pulse—Instrument for measuring rate at which pulse-type signals occur.

Reactance—An electrical characteristic, which impedes the flow of alternating current because of the inductance and capacitance in a circuit. Measured in ohms.

Rectifier—An electron tube, selenium or copper-oxide device, or crystal employed in such a manner as to convert alternating current into unidirectional current.

Refractometer—Instrument using measurement of index of refraction of a substance for analytical purposes.

Regulated power supply—A power supply device containing means for maintaining constant voltage or constant current under changing load conditions.

Resistance—The opposition to an electric current characteristic of a circuit element or medium.

Resistor—An electrical component which offers resistance to the flow of current.

Resonance—A condition in a circuit containing inductance and capacitance in which the inductive reactance is equal and opposite to the capacitive reactance. This condition occurs at but one frequency for a given fixed circuit and the circuit is said to be "at resonance."

Sawtooth voltage—A voltage that varies between two values in a manner to provide a waveform pattern resembling the teeth of a saw. (Also called *ramp voltage.*)

Schematic diagram—A diagram of the general scheme of an electrical circuit, with graphical symbols representing components.

Selectivity—The degree to which a circuit can accept the signals of one frequency while rejecting those of all others.

Sensitivity—The degree to which a device can reproduce weak signals with satisfactory gain.

Shunt—(1) A resistor connected across the terminals of a meter to increase the meter range by allowing part of the current to by-pass the meter. (2) An electrical component or part connected in parallel with another component, or part.

Signal—The intelligence, message, or effect conveyed in electronic applications.

Signal-noise ratio—The ratio of the magnitude of the desired signal to that of undesired noise signal.

Signal tracing–The technique of tracing a signal through each stage in order to locate a faulty stage.

Spectrophotometer–Analytical instrument which relies on selective absorption of light by specimen for identification.

Stethoscope, electronic–Electronic amplifier of sounds within body. Selective controls permit tuning for low heart tones or high pulmonary tones; has auxiliary output for recording or viewing audio patterns.

Strain gauge–Device for measuring the expansion or contraction of an object. Comprised of wires that change resistance with expansion or contraction.

Switch–A mechanical device for opening and closing an electrical circuit.

Telemetry equipment system–System for transmitting data acquired at one location to a different location for recording or display.

Tetrode–An electron tube with four electrodes: a cathode (electron emitter), a plate (electron collector), and usually two grids for controlling the flow of electrons.

Thermal conductivity detector–Device for indicating heat flux through metal, gas, solution, etc.

Thermistor–A temperature sensitive resistor.

Thermocouple–Temperature transducer comprised of a closed circuit made of two different metals. If the two junctions are at different temperatures, an electromotive force is developed which is proportional to the temperature difference between the junctions.

Thermometer, electronic–Device that measures and/or records temperature electronically.

Thyratron–A hot cathode, gas-filled tube used as a discharge device. Nonconducting until grid potential ionizes the gas within the tube.

Transducer–Device that changes one form of energy to another, *eg,* pressure, temperature, pulse to electrical signal.

Transducer, Doppler ultrasonic–Device that detects motion by a shift in the frequency of reflected sound (Doppler effect).

Transformer–Coils mounted on a common support so that the magnetic lines of force produced by alternating current or by pulsating direct current flowing through one coil induce a corresponding alternating voltage in the other coil.

Transistor–An electron device utilizing properties of semiconductors (such as germanium) as detectors, amplifiers, and oscillators of electric currents.

Triode—An electron tube with three electrodes: a cathode (electron emitter), a place (electron collector), and a control grid. Used in amplifier oscillator circuits.

Ultrasonic—Frequencies which lie just above the audible range (sometimes called *supersonic*).

Ultrasonic generator—Device that produces signals of ultrasonic frequency (> 20 KHz).

Ultrasonic probe—Rod for directing ultrasonic force. Used in disintegration or foreign body location applications.

Ultrasonic scanner—Ultrasonic diagnostic instrument for visualizing tissue/organ interfaces and presenting cross-sectional images.

Variable capacitor—A capacitor, the capacitance of which can be changed by varying the useful area of the capacitor plates.

Variable resistor—A wire-wound or composition resistor, the value of which may be changed.

Varistor—A device which has the property of changing resistance when influenced by the voltage applied.

Vectorcardiograph—Instrument for determining magnitude and direction along x, y and z axes of cardiac signals acting during heart cycle.

Volt (v)—The basic unit of voltage or electromotive force.

Watt (w)—The unit of electric power.

Wavelength—The distance between successive peaks of the same polarity in a wave. Corresponds to the distance traveled by the wave in one cycle.

X-ray apparatus, medical—Equipment for producing penetrating X-radiation (radiation with wavelength between 10^{-7} and 10^{-9} cm), directing the radiation through objects to be examined, and detecting the transmitted radiation by fluorescence, photography, or ionization effects.

X-ray therapy apparatus, radiotherapy apparatus—High energy X-ray equipment used for radiation-destruction of malignant tumors or for radiation-treatment of skin conditions, etc.

index